ReMission Possible

Yours, If You Choose To Accept It

Barby Ingle

San Tan Valley, Arizona, USA

ReMission Possible

Yours, If You Choose To Accept It

ISBN-13: 978-0615452227
ISBN-10: 0615452221

Printed in the United States of America.

Author Barby Ingle
Editor Ray Bilkie
Photography by Ken Taylor and Matthew Henschke

Introduction

The two most asked questions I get regarding Reflex Sympathetic Dystrophy are: is there a cure and will Ketamine help? Patients are looking for specific information on Ketamine treatments, the nuts and bolts, not just an overview. Finally, *ReMission Possible* is a book that addresses both issues!

According to the Webster Dictionary, remission is a lessening of the symptoms of a disease, or their temporary reduction or disappearance.

ReMission Possible shows in great detail the process of treatment and remission in Barby's journey. My idea of what remission is and is not has been changed forever. I have known many people with RSD[1] that have gone into remission and back to their old lives. They prefer not to discuss the experience or share the journey with others. This is an important topic and I am glad someone has finally tackled it.

It is important to know you may get worse before getting better and you may not totally regain your exact former life. It may be a slightly different version of our former self. Not worse, just different.

Ketamine treatments have helped Barby tremendously. It is not the first line of defense for the treatment of Reflex Sympathetic Dystrophy. However, for many people who

---

[1] Reflex Sympathetic Dystrophy has had over 20 name designations since the Civil War. Other names include: Polytrauma; Reflex Neurovascular Dystrophy, RND; Algoneurodystrophy; Sudeck's Atrophy; Regional Pain Syndrome; Complex Regional Pain Syndrome, CRPS; Reflex Sympathetic Dystrophy, RSD; Shoulder-Hand Syndrome; Post Traumatic Dystrophy; Painful Post Traumatic Dystrophy; Painful Post-Traumatic Osteoporosis; and Transient Migratory Osteoporosis.

have tried multiple treatments with little or no success, Ketamine is worth considering. I chose not to try it and one of the reasons was the lack of detailed information regarding the process. This book fills in the blanks.

Talking to your doctor is very important. Equally important is reading a book like this from the patient's perspective.

Trudy Thomas
Host of "Living with HOPE" radio show
The Body, Mind and Spirit Network

I consider it a privilege to be one of the first individuals to have read this masterful anecdote about one person's victory over Reflex Sympathetic Dystrophy through IV Infusion therapy.

I am immediately drawn to the message of hope and optimism Barby has so carefully created in this uplifting and wonderful story of trial, tribulation and eventual triumph. I have seen firsthand many aspects of Barby's struggle. Barby takes us through her great efforts to find a good social balance and not push our limits that are still present after remission too far.

Barby's ability to get others to listen helps our cause with insurance companies and medical professionals who choose not to cover these important treatments. This book highlights some of the aspects that refute these third-party influences that work to fight against paying or offering this possible relief to patients.

Jodi Dragon, Executive Board
Power of Pain Foundation

Acknowledgements

Throughout 2009 and 2010, I began a new journey. I want to thank so many people who were in my life at this time and helped me get to where I am today:

God

PA Healthcare Team
- Dr. Schwartzman, Carol, Lynn, and the rest of Dr. Schwartzman's Staff
- Nurse Colleen at Drexel Hospital

To My Family
- My Husband Ken
- My Father Jim
- My Sister Marby and Her Husband Brian and Jellybean
- My Brother Jimmy, His Wife Jennifer and both Nephews Jon Hall and Jacob
- My Brother Timmy, and His Wife Sarah, And Johan! Thank You (For Putting A Smile On My Face, Even In The Worst Of Times)!
- My Mother Chriss

People Who Helped Me With Fundraising
- Cheerleader #2- Shelley Moyer
- Tom Deluca
- Sara Schlossman
- Julia Beall
- All of the Other Donors who Helped Me Raise the Funding To Get the IV-Infusion Therapy Which Put Me Into Remission

AZ Healthcare Team
- Dr. Steven Siwek For Administering My Boosters
- Dr. Matthew Hummel

Best Friends / Emotional Support Team

- Barb Black
- Jodi Dragon
- Kyle Kendrix
- Patty Parkhurst
- Ray Bilkie
- Thomas "Santa" SanNicholas

Other Patients and Friends

- Colonel Douglas Strand, USAF: A Fellow RSD'er Who Is Fighting For A Disability Rating For Reflex Sympathetic Dystrophy In The Military. Thanks To You And Vivian For Letting Me Help You Out On This Important Issue
- Dominick Spatafora
- Danielle Freudenheim

Media

- The Staff At AZTV Ch. 3 and ABC Ch. 15 Both in Arizona For Putting Me On TV To Tell My Story And Spread Awareness
- Trudy Thomas For Having Me On Her Radio Show Multiple Times and Giving Such High Praise To Her Listeners Of "Living With Hope" To My First Book
- Vicky Carmona For Having Me On Her Radio Show "Sunday Sunrise" Multiple Times and All The Support Over The Years With Awareness Issues

No Category:

- Pfizer For Making Ketamine

Thank You So Much To All Of The People Who Have Made This Process And My Life Great, Shown Me Love And Support the Whole Way Through, Both Before and After Remission. Many Blessings and Prayers to All!

- Barby *\o/* (shake the poms)

Contents

1

OFF I GO

"Off I Go Is Where I Land."
Greg Laswell

This is a book for chronically ill patients who want to understand what remission brings. A lot of people think remission means: done, I get my life back now. Most people do not realize that remission is a new experience all in itself. This book is good for the chronically ill, pain patients, family members, caregivers, healthcare professionals and the public. One in three people in the United States are affected with a condition that causes pain, so it is bound to affect you or someone you know. Until you feel the pain, it is difficult to understand the challenges it brings on. Whether physical or mental, pain can, and will consume you if you allow it to. Only the patient can begin the process of healing. My hope is that through my speaking engagements and books, I will inspire your eventual transformation of great positivity in life and one filled with hope. Healing starts from within. No pill or drug can duplicate the power within you. Here's to turning your pain to power!

Whether you have been in remission or are still dreaming of it, know that it will be a new chapter in life, and expecting the same life you always knew before your condition set in may not be so realistic. This does not mean it will not be fulfilling, positive, hopeful and a great experience. Chronic conditions such as the neurological condition I have, Reflex Sympathetic Dystrophy, are lifelong changers. The hope and success of remission is still yet another journey.

I have been battling a neurological condition for 8+ years now. Reflex Sympathetic Dystrophy is a progressive condition and needs to be treated early so that disability does not take over. I know firsthand how hard it is to continue looking for relief, answers, and coming up against healthcare professionals who blow you off, or do not believe what you are describing could actually be what you are experiencing. Many healthcare professionals will try to connect the pain back to some traumatic experience in your past. You may have gotten over the past years ago, but they do not have answers, so it is an easy way out for why they cannot fix you. Over the years, while searching for a cure, I have also grown emotionally and spiritually. Even after seeing over a hundred healthcare professionals, getting major surgeries I did not need, having complications such as internal bleeding, medication interactions, kidney stones, tumors growing in my mouth, and so much more, I did not give up or give in! I was tested physically and mentally to my limits and realized they are past the bounds I placed on myself. I am stronger than I ever knew. I had to become the chief of staff of my own medical team. If I can do it, anyone can.

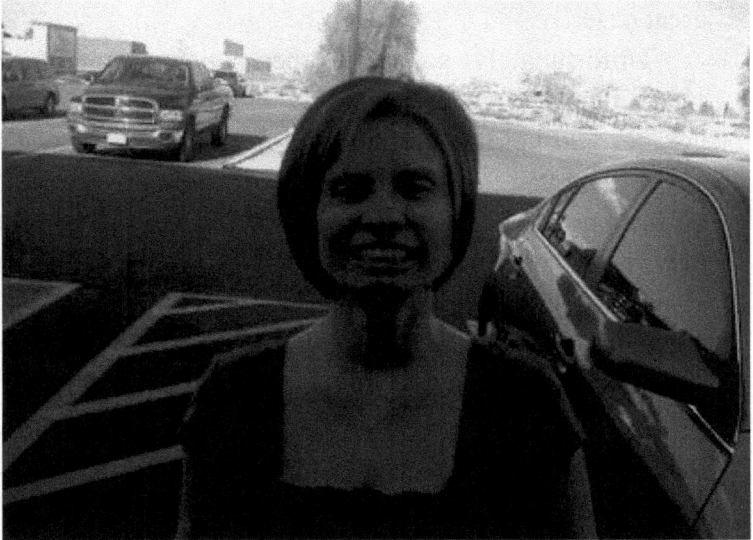

Barby on her way to a doctor's appointment 2009

The healthcare system is not what we are led to believe as we grow up. Doctors are not miracle workers in themselves. They are human just as we all are. We call doctors who treat patients practicing physicians for a reason. People look up to their doctors and put total faith in them. I know I did in the beginning. I have learned through my experience with so many of my own treating doctors and through volunteering with the Power of Pain

Foundation that I am responsible for myself, just as you are for yourself. I also learned that doctors study a particular field of medicine. Just because they are neurologists does not mean they can treat both multiple sclerosis and RSD. Each doctor gets a small variety of a medical field and then finds a part of a specialty that they love and work on with great ease.

Unfortunately, so many other patients experience my story. I now want to share my knowledge to lower this number and help those going through the health system at any level. I had to learn the hard way and now want to pass on my knowledge to give hope and answers to patients so they do not have to go through the same. By speaking out about my journey, I am not spewing complaints. I am presenting how I have overcome the challenges presented to me through different experiences.

For the readers who do not know or understand what Reflex Sympathetic Dystrophy is, here is a short explanation. Anyone can get it. Any age, any race. The hallmark of the condition is severe burning pain. However, all of the other symptoms that are involved with Reflex Sympathetic Dystrophy and how it physically affects the patient is not discussed much, but can be just as debilitating and progressive. Unlike other chronic conditions (ie; diabetes, cancer, multiple sclerosis), there does not seem to be any urgency on Reflex Sympathetic Dystrophy or finding a cure. This condition has been studied and researched for over 150 years, yet much of society and healthcare field professionals haven't heard of it or don't know what is involved and just how complex it really is.

This is in spite of the statistics of prevalence being in the millions with a high estimate of 6,000,000. The Reflex Sympathetic Dystrophy Syndrome Association places statistics at an estimated 50,000-78,000 new cases developing each year in the United States. People do not typically die from it physically, although doctors have told me you can die from pain. Many patients do however go into depression and have to learn to live with constant pain and neurological symptoms. Some cannot handle this, and unfortunately, a percentage will commit suicide just to stop the torture. Reflex Sympathetic Dystrophy is a progressive condition that involves the sympathetic nervous system, reflexive body actions, limbic system, immune system, vision, hearing, dystonia and dystrophy of muscle and bone. Some are lucky (if you can call it that) in the fact that they are only affected in one extremity or that they go into remission. My Reflex Sympathetic Dystrophy started with burning in my face, neck and shoulder, but with all of the complications over the years, it now affects my entire body including my heart, intestines, swallowing, immune system and so much more. Reflex Sympathetic Dystrophy has recently been found to be a neuroinflammatory disease.

What is neuroinflammation and why does it cause such severe burning pain even when there seems to be no injury? Let me explain as simply as I can. Say you sprain your ankle. Your ankle then hurts, swells, discolors, and the pain limits use. The swelling occurs because of "healing" chemicals that move into the affected area and work to heal any damage. In a typical person this process is successful, and the healing chemicals trigger another set of chemicals to take the healing chemical away, thus the swelling and discoloration go away. With Reflex Sympathetic Dystrophy, the second set of chemicals is not activated. Without that healing process functioning correctly, the prolonged neuroinflammation becomes chronic and activates what we know as glial in your spine and brain. Many specialists in Reflex Sympathetic Dystrophy have said that there is a window of six to nine months to correct this healing process. Others say it is shorter or longer. Nonetheless, this poor healing process "changes your spine and brain" and essentially turns on your pain signals and activates your glia. This often-permanent activation is Reflex Sympathetic Dystrophy.

Glials are small nerve cells that fire off about every two minutes looking for any threats to the body. This is part of your fight or flight system. Glial cells are sometimes called neuroglia or simply glia. They are non-neuronal cells that maintain homeostasis, form myelin, and provide support and protection for the brain's neurons. Glia is a Greek word meaning glue. In the human brain, there is roughly one glia for every neuron with a ratio of about two neurons for every three glia in the cerebral gray matter.[2]

The four main functions of glial cells are to surround neurons and hold them in place, supply nutrients and oxygen to neurons, insulate one neuron from another, to destroy pathogens and remove dead neurons. They also

---

[2] Azevedo FA, Carvalho LR, Grinberg LT, Farfel JM, Ferretti RE, Leite RE, Jacob Filho W, Lent R, Herculano-Houzel S. (2009). Equal numbers of neuronal and nonneuronal cells make the human brain an isometrically scaled-up primate brain. J Comp Neurol. 513(5):532-41

modulate neurotransmission.[3] Therefore, glia is a lot more than just the "glue" of the nervous system. Another well-known item, narcotics, also activates glia. I will go into why this is important in an upcoming chapter.

One of the recent theories I have heard is 'priming of the nervous system'. I can best explain it how Dr. Linda Watkins explained it at a pain conference last year. Let's say that someone slaps you unexpectedly. Your body reacts with a fight or flight response. Then down the road a few months, maybe a year, someone slaps you. Now your fight or flight response is on guard for the situation. It wants to be ready to protect you if any new situation occurs where you may be slapped again. The 'slap' is any trauma. The first can be a torn ligament or broken bone or even a paper cut. The second can be just as big as or smaller than the first incident. The first incident causes the priming. The second confirms the risk, even if there is not one; the body's system is 'on' just in case. Now this is only one theory and it is relatively new, but it makes a lot of sense to me.

Recently, I was speaking with a friend who is a research doctor. He was explaining to me that a study was recently completed in Liverpool that shows Reflex Sympathetic Dystrophy is an autoimmune disease. A Reflex Sympathetic Dystrophy patient in Canada, who was recently sick, further evidenced this. The doctor put her on an antibiotic and her RSD symptoms disappeared. Once she was well, they took her off the antibiotic and the symptoms

[3] FEBS J. 2008 Jul;275(14):3514-26.d- Amino acids in the brain: d-serine in neurotransmission and neurodegeneration. Wolosker H, Dumin E, Balan L, Foltyn VN.

returned. Her doctor put her back on the medication and the symptoms disappeared again. This gave the researchers something to base their studies on. My friend stated that there would soon be a blood test that can tell a person if they have the antigen in their body. Once they isolate the exact one, they will be able to create an antidote or antibiotic that will target this specifically. This is big news. It is great in the progress of finding a cure.

How is RSD different from other autoimmune conditions? One difference is that the RSD can be in you lying dormant for your whole life and may never affect you negatively. Something your body perceives as a trauma triggers the attack. I can see it also having a negative effect on court cases. RSD is hard enough to explain to a jury now. When the defense throws in that it is autoimmune, I can see a jury becoming confused on what to believe. People would not normally sue if they caught lime disease from a tick bite. This process is easier to explain to the court case participants in states with the 'egg shell law'. Imagine an egg with cracks in it. The egg is still whole, but has some issues. Once something breaks the shell, you cannot put the egg back exactly the way it was prior to the trauma. The egg breaking is the trauma that changes the egg forever, just as an accident or injury is the trauma that changes us forever.

A more positive thought is how this can affect the military. Soldiers are developing Reflex Sympathetic Dystrophy at high rates. If they were able to do this blood test at the time of entry into the armed forces they could screen out potential cases of Reflex Sympathetic Dystrophy development, atleast from military injuries for these people. If you knew that you had a propensity for Reflex Sympathetic Dystrophy development, you could live your life a little differently, lowering the chances of a trauma that may change your life.

****

Here is my time, my chance, my everything, to possibly reverse what I have been living with since 2002. My excitement is great, along with the rest of my family. My regular treating doctors are not so optimistic, but are not discouraging either. I believe deep down that Ketamine infusions will put me into remission. I have hope that other doctors around the country will begin to do the protocol that Dr. Schwartzman is using, and more RSD'ers will reap the benefits sooner. I know my doctor here in Arizona, Dr. Steven Siwek, is working with a local hospital to provide it, and in the meantime, he is providing me IV-Ketamine boosters as an outpatient, using Dr. Schwartzman's protocol. I am going to tell you about my story as it has continued since my first published book *RSD in Me!* and about my experience of remission.

Postponed, But Why?

February 2009
The anticipation of this journey is coming to a head. One of the leading RSD specialists in the United States is Dr. Robert Schwartzman. I have heard others say that their

wait was up to five years to get in to see him. I have been on Dr. Schwartzman's waiting list for IV-Ketamine infusions since 2007. Here I am, two years later, leaving in a few days for my appointment in Pennsylvania. This procedure can be life changing. I have so many friends that the infusion therapy helped, so my hopes are high and my belief is soaring.

Since 2002, when my auto accident occurred, all I want is to get better and get my life back. All that has happened up to this point is that I have become weaker physically, and my entire body is now affected, including my heart, intestines, immune system and more. The neurological condition, Reflex Sympathetic Dystrophy, is a stress producer on your body as well as your mind. It affects all aspects of life just as all chronic illnesses do. The strain of financial stress, marital pressure, family expectations and loss of social life can be devastating if you do not keep your life challenges in perspective.

March 2009

I was suppose be in Pennsylvania in February to see Dr. Schwartzman, but my appointment was moved to March 30, 2009. I fly out later this month and will be out on the east coast for about a month. I am saddened by the delay but know that there is good reason. Others still have years to wait, so I cannot complain.

Coincidently, at the time my appointment was moved back a month, Dr. Schwartzman was on national news because of complications that occurred with one of his patients in Germany who was undergoing the IV-Ketamine coma treatment. From news reports, I found the problem was not with the IV-Ketamine, but rather the female patient had the MRSA infection, and she had it even before leaving the United States. The virus caused complications and additional bills that her family was not expecting to incur. I still feel fully confident in the process and am moving ahead. I understand that people are upset with the process and don't understand why it costs so much, or why many doctors are not choosing to perform this treatment that the FDA approved and proven to be effective in many Neuropathy pain patients.

I know not all patients respond to Ketamine treatments, but this is a noninvasive procedure that has three levels of treatment depending on what state you are in with all of the neurological symptoms and burning pain.

Going For IV-Infusion Therapy, Got None.

Dr. Schwartzman saw me on March 30. He also had seven other internists with him during the exam. I learned a lot. The bad news I received that day was that I am full body Reflex Sympathetic Dystrophy. I am experiencing sympathetically independent pain vs. sympathetically mediated pain. It is a lot more difficult to treat SIP and his suggestion is now that I go for Ketamine coma.

As it turns out, I was not going for the infusion. I was going for a consult. I am on a waiting list that could take just months or up to two years. I thought that I could see Dr. Schwartzman, have a few days of testing and then begin outpatient Ketamine treatments. After his consult and neurological test, it was evident that this plan was not going to work and that I needed much more invasive treatment than I ever imagined. So, I headed home to see Ken.

****

I came home to Arizona and have a lot of thinking to do in preparation for my treatments. I am not sure what I want to do. I have been depressed since the visit with Dr. Schwartzman. I have always been strong mentally while dealing with the challenges of Reflex Sympathetic Dystrophy. This time, I was having great trouble getting over the news I heard. It took me over a month to come out of the depression. In the meantime, I am on the waiting list for the coma and inpatient ICU infusions. Whichever comes up first is what I will do. It is weird to go through this process. I feel like I am on a waiting list for a kidney that is going to save my life. Actually, I am just waiting for a bed in an ICU unit, in one of the only hospital in the United States doing this procedure, or a bed in a Mexican hospital to have the coma treatment. I found out that Medicare covers 80% of the infusions done in the United States but I will have to raise $40,000 for the coma procedure. At this point, I am leaning towards the infusion procedure and will then do the coma if maximum results are not achieved. Dr. Schwartzman thought that the coma could prove to give me 100% effectiveness vs. the infusion that is estimated at 80% effectiveness at best. I have a thick packet to read through over the next few weeks. I will give updates of what I am learning. My wait for the coma may be up to two years and I return to Pennsylvania for more testing in mid May. This time, my husband gets to go with me.

Meeting Dr. Schwartzman

So, what happened during the appointment? When I arrived at Dr. Schwartzman's office, I was excited. I was with my sister and her husband who live in Virginia. Ken did not come with me this time because he had to work. When I start the infusion, I will be isolated for the week anyway and he would be sitting here bored. My family only lives a few hours away from Pennsylvania so it was an easy drive after a long flight across the country. I am hurting all over and many of my symptoms are flaring. I have many types of pain going on right now: burning, stabbing, electric, shooting, deep, surface, bone. I am dizzy from it. Feeling nauseated does not help either.

My name is finally called and my sister and I go the examining room. The nurse is very nice and asks all the right questions. We told her that we'd like to document everything and asked if it would it be okay if we taped the exam. She did not see a problem with it but said the doctor would have the final say. I had also brought the doctor a copy of my book, *RSD in Me!* I was very excited to give it to him, since I spoke about him in one of the chapters. We had previously met in Las Vegas during a conference for the American Academy of Pain Management.

When he had walked into the room to see me, his first words were, "Now she has Reflex Sympathetic Dystrophy.

Anyone should be able to see it at first glance." Not all of the doctors who had previously treated me could recognize the symptoms that I had Reflex Sympathetic Dystrophy, and their knowledge was limited. He then began pointing out all of the symptoms, or as I saw it, the flaws I had from the Reflex Sympathetic Dystrophy. He knew things before I even said anything. Actually, I did not know to say anything, because I did not know all that was involved.

They had me put on a gown when I came into the room. The doctors saw the blanching from head to toe. From my face to my feet, I had discoloration. I never paid that much attention to how bad it had gotten over the years; maybe because it happened over time. I took pictures of it over the last few years, but did not know it meant that Reflex Sympathetic Dystrophy was in that area. The more severe burning pain was on the right side of my body. Although I had all the other types of pain on the left side, the symptoms of atrophy and coordination were not as bad. I greeted and passed him my book. He recognized me from the conference in Vegas and he seemed to recall my case. I was worse now than I was two years ago. He thanked me for my book and then I introduced him to my sister and he continued with the exam.

When he began to do the neurological testing on both sides, I felt the pain. The right side was worse, but the left side was definitely affected. He discussed me being diagnosed incorrectly by my other doctors with Thoracic Outlet Syndrome near the beginning of this process and having my rib removed twice with my other doctors. He guessed correctly that I had been diagnosed with TMJ because of the facial pain and that I was having issues with my thyroid. He remarked about the sweating, swelling in areas, asked about my low-grade fevers, Horner's syndrome and more. He noted the atrophy in my hands, arms, legs, feet, face, back and the dystonia in my hands and feet. By discussed, I mean he discussed it with the other doctors. He hardly spoke to me.

Next, he had me do neurological tests. An easy one that you can do right now only involves your hand. Take the tip of your pointer finger and tap it to the tip of your thumb as many times and as fast as you can. I thought that I did it very well, especially on the left hand. He explained how I did it, awkward and slow, was another symptom. I did not understand, so he showed me. He could tap his fingers so fast that it looked like I was going in slow motion. Since then, I ask others to do the same thing. I am amazed that I cannot go that fast no matter how hard I try.

He watched me smile, had me stick my tongue out and then asked me if I have trouble swallowing and does my voice go in and out sometimes. I said, "Yes, how did you know?" He said that the Reflex Sympathetic Dystrophy was affecting my throat and intestines.

I had been diagnosed with gastrointestinal ischemia a few years back. The hospitalist that performed the tests said there is a section of my intestines that is getting little to no blood. I did not understand just how it was related to the Reflex Sympathetic Dystrophy until this visit when I learned that with Reflex Sympathetic Dystrophy you have vascular constriction. Vascular constriction makes it difficult to get an IV line inserted or even do blood tests. I never realized that the constriction could also affect organs. I thought I was just eating too quickly or being lazy when I choked on food. I did not know why my voice changed or why I would lose it sometimes. The Reflex Sympathetic Dystrophy affected even my nails and hair growth. He was spot on with everything. He added that whiplash or brachia plexus injuries are a leading cause of upper extremity Reflex Sympathetic Dystrophy. With all of my additional traumas and surgeries, the Reflex Sympathetic Dystrophy had spread.

My sister was videotaping and he saw her shaking her head, as he would name off symptoms and issues I had been going through. He stopped, turned to her and asked, "Why are you shaking your head?" She replied, "Everything you are saying is correct. Barby has all of those symptoms." His reply to that was, "You don't know anything. If I gave you a test right now you would not pass it." It was very cold of him, but I can understand where it was coming from. He has worked with Reflex Sympathetic Dystrophy patients, thousands of them, over the last forty years. She is just a sister of a patient with Reflex Sympathetic Dystrophy. He had seven other doctors in the room that he was trying to teach and more patients to attend to after me.

Dr. Schwartzman made a big deal about this: narcotics! He asked if I was taking any. I said ultram when needed and, rarely, morphine. He told me that if I wanted to do the Ketamine treatments and have it work, I needed to get off all narcotics, even ultram. He also told me to stop radio frequency ablations. When I come back to undergo the IV-

16

Ketamine, they want me in the most raw form, so the system would reboot better. Through his research and working with so many patients, he apparently realized that patients who are on narcotics do not have the same results as people who stop them. Since then, I have learned that narcotics also set off glia. Therefore, if you are taking narcotics and have Reflex Sympathetic Dystrophy you are causing yourself more problems physically, although, you may not care because they also help you mentally escape the pain you are feeling. Dull it, so to say. In addition, he needs you off the narcotics because the glia has a Ketamine receptor. In non-technical language, the Ketamine turns off the fight or flight response. If you take a narcotic, you are just turning it back on.

Now, I was ready to hear, "We will do testing over the next few days and then start Ketamine next week." Instead, I got something I never thought I was going to hear.

Sometime near the end of the exam, Dr. Schwartzman was talking to the student doctors about me. He said, "The only thing that will help this patient 100% is the coma treatment." I was in shock. I thought I was going to be getting an outpatient infusion therapy for ten days and then start boosters. I began to tear up. I kept telling myself not to cry. It is never good to cry at the medical doctor's office. I wanted to be taken seriously and be strong. As soon as they left the room, tears flowed down my face. The nurse said she would be right back with all of the instructions and scripts that he was giving me. When she came back into the exam room, she informed us that Dr. Schwartzman was not comfortable with the videotaping and that we needed to erase it. I would have had my sister taking notes if we knew that; we thought we were going to have a videotape of it and there would be no need to take notes. Once we got into the car, my sister told me that she had not erased it. So, we have it for private use and reference, but I cannot make it public.

I did not have any idea of the issues that were involved with Reflex Sympathetic Dystrophy and that I had many of the symptoms. I am now thinking these are going to be some long two years.

2

TESTING, TESTING!

*"I believe life is constantly testing us for our level
of commitment, and life's greatest rewards are reserved
for those who demonstrate a never-ending commitment
to act until they achieve. This level of resolve can
move mountains, but it must be constant and consistent.
As simplistic as this may sound, it is still the common
denominator separating those who live their dreams
from those who live in regret."*
Tony Robbins

Now it is time to prepare. I am going to undergo testing
on my heart, lungs, kidneys, liver, x-rays, quantitative
sensory testing, and psychological testing. Some of the
testing I can do in Arizona. A few of the tests need to be
completed with Dr. Schwartzman's specialist.

They have to be sure I am physically and mentally
ready for the Ketamine treatments. There can be issues so
they rule out people who have problems in any of these

areas. I do not see myself having trouble in any of the areas, but we will soon find out. I have my dates set for returning to Pennsylvania in May and have begun my testing that can be done here in Arizona.

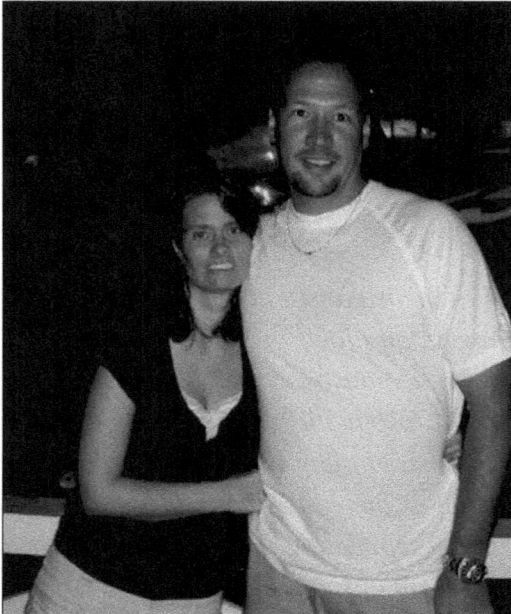

Barby and Ken (her husband) 2008

Psychological Evaluation

May 2009

I flew to Pennsylvania for my Monday testing appointments this past Saturday. I was also notified that I was chosen for American Idol finale tickets on Friday afternoon, as I was getting ready to go fly out to

Pennsylvania. The American Idol finale is this coming Wednesday. Last year I was unable to attend due to a visit with my lawyers and I really wanted to find a way to attend this year. It is looking like I will not be able to attend.

Sunday, I rested in Philadelphia at the hotel with my husband to recover from the traveling. Monday morning I reported to Dr. Schwartzman's office and met with two neuropsychology doctors. During the first hour and a half, I was asked questions about my medical history, how I feel about my situation and then some cognitive testing. It all went great. Then, I spent time with the neuropsychiatrist discussing the results and the upcoming Ketamine procedure. Ken was able to come in for this part. I then went in the waiting room for another hour and a half. I completed a personality test that was multiple-choice. By this time, my pain levels were through the roof and I was on the verge of vomiting, so Ken did all the writing for me. He is the greatest.

Ken ran and got us lunch from the Quizno's across the street from the hospital and doctor's office as soon as we were done with the testing. There were about 300 questions we had to get through. The neuropsychiatrist went over my answers while Ken was gone. He came out to the lobby and let me know that I was cleared for Ketamine on the psychological part and that I was in normal range for what I was going through.

As I was finishing my lunch, the next doctor came to get me for autonomic sensory testing (QST-AST).

Sensory Testing

The room was like a closet, very small. There was so much equipment in there the doctor had trouble moving it in place at times. I was nervous about how painful these tests would be, but it went fine. First test was a hot/cold test. This test was performed on both of my hands and feet. The device was about 2x1x1 black box, probably made out of metal. It is put on two places on each extremity. The test was neat to complete. The doctor heated and cooled the box and it could instantly turn back to room temperature. On my right hand, one of the cold times, I could not hold back from yelling from the pain. I started to tear up. He said I was very sensitive to touch and cold which I already knew. This test was used instead of a nerve biopsy. The doctor said it was actually more accurate and told them more information than the biopsy would have.

Then, we did a laser picture, it is like a thermogram, but it is more accurate from what I understood. I asked for copies of the picture and it will be a few weeks until I can get it. This laser machine drew out line by line a picture of my thermal image. It was so apparent where the Reflex Sympathetic Dystrophy was from this image. I have been to the Smithsonian Institute in Washington DC where they have a thermogram. You could see the difference with me on that screen but it was not all over as this one was. Still, I drew a crowd at the museum because no one else's scan looked like mine. That scanner was nowhere as sensitive as the one currently being used in Dr. Schwartzman's office. Unfortunately, I am guessing that most people who do the laser thermogram testing for Ketamine clearance have results similar to mine and it would not be a big deal.

After that, we did a temperature test. He used this handheld thermometer and touched each finger and other parts of my palms and feet to take measurements. They were close in measurements, but with bodywide Reflex Sympathetic Dystrophy that is reasonably expected. I remember when it was just in my arm and it was two to five degrees colder than the other arm at all times.

Next was a vibration test. I thought it was going to hurt. All it enitialed was a small black box with a sensor the size of a dime sticking up. I put my index finger and then my pinky on the sensor and he would turn it up. As soon as I felt it, I would tell him and he cut it off.

The final test was a coordination test. You can try it. Take a keyboard and put your thumb below the space bar and your index finger on the key. You might have to have someone hold the keyboard for you. Have someone time sixty seconds while you hit the bar as many times as you can. On my left hand, I got just over seventy and my right was around thirty. He said that the average for a healthly person is 150-170. I thought I was doing well until he said that. I asked him to show me what normal would look like and he did the test. I was amazed at how quick he was. Then the testing was over.

The sensory testing doctor said he was done early because I went through the test so fast due to the sensitivity. I went through the test fast because as soon as you feel it, your measurement is done and you move on.

Ken and I then rested for the remainder of the day and

prepared to fly home at 4 A.M. EST (1 A.M. our time) to Arizona.

We landed in AZ around 11 A.M. Ken surprised me and said we were flying on from Arizona to Los Angeles if I could handle it. I decided to fly through the pain and head to California for American Idol. I was hurting already, might as well have this great life experience. The finale was great and worth the extra pain. It was a once in a lifetime event and one of the best memories of life I have.

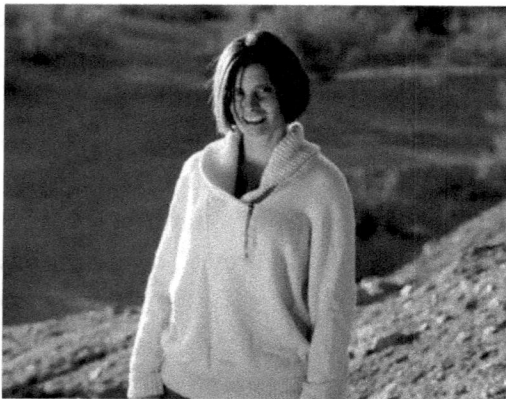

Barby Ingle 2011

Overall, the trip was successful. I do have to get one additional cardiac test done here in Arizona before I can be scheduled for the Ketamine. My EKG test I had in Arizona before I left came back with an abnormal finding and I have to have more testing. I see my pain doctor in two weeks and my first fundraiser is coming up in June. I am full of hope for the future and happy I was able to have a good life experience in the mist of all of the challenges.

American Idol or Bust!

We got great seats. You would not believe the "stars" that were right around us and who I met. To name a few: Janice Dickinson, many of the past idols, Heather Locklear, the Black Eyed Peas and Billy Bush. Unfortunately, I did not recognize Fergie until she was on stage to perform. I had given her directions on how to get back stage without realizing with whom I was speaking. The other stars were on the red carpet and then just went into the event with the rest of us like regular people. People hung out in the lobby until seating began.

In the lobby, I was walking past Billy Bush and said, "Hey, Billy Bush, nice to meet you." He was very approachable and friendly. He shook my left hand as no one shakes my right. I told him I follow him on Twitter and he said they took away his Blackberry so he could not tweet from the show. They did not let phones or cameras in, so we left ours in the car. The person behind us snuck one in and we noticed him on the phone. We asked him to take a picture of us and e-mail it. So he did.

The show began and it was one surprise after another. On the last commercial break, Ken said, "Let's go meet Paula." We were sitting left center and by the time we got out of our row, Paula had gone backstage, so there was no chance. I was very scared of the security too. I did not want to look like a stalker, but I wanted to give her a Reflex Sympathetic Dystrophy awareness bracelet from our foundation. Since she was not there, I saw Billy Bush sitting about eight rows down, got brave, and approached him again.

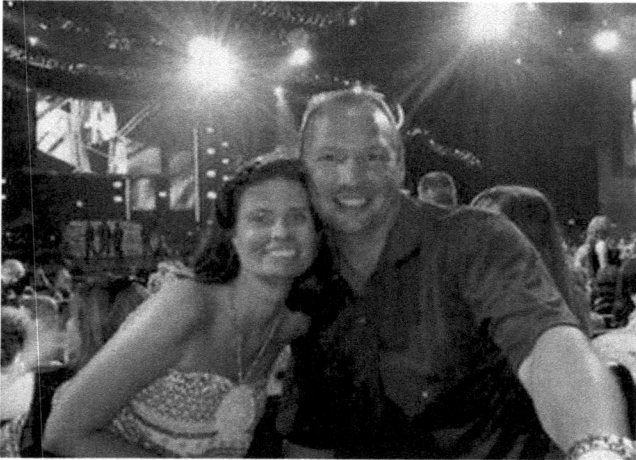

Barby and Ken at American Idol 2009

I asked if he was going to the after party and he said yes. I told him that I would like him to give Paula the bracelet and that we both had Reflex Sympathetic Dystrophy. It did not register with him at first, so I said "pain condition" and he remembered. I told him I sent a copy of my book to Paula a few weeks ago and that I wanted to give her the Reflex Sympathetic Dystrophy awareness bracelet. He seemed impressed that I wrote a book.

In the meantime, a security guard came up to me and started to grab me to tell me to sit down. Ken jumped in and said, "Do not touch her," and the guard turned around. Billy went to reach out and touch me too. Ken put his hand out to keep him from touching me and said, "Do not touch her. She has a pain condition." I just kept talking; I knew this was my only chance.

The producers announced 30 seconds to air over the loud system. Needing to hurry back to my seat, I said to Billy, "Please tell her this is from Barby (like the doll)." I thanked him and started to turn back to walk to my seat. Then he said, "You've got your wish!" I was so excited. Even if she does not contact me, I am happy to know that Billy would pass on my message.

I wish we could have stayed longer, but by then Ken had to leave because of his work early next morning and I was fine with it, my body in total pain. Still, I am happy with this experience and will always cherish it!

How's My Heart Ticking?

May 2009

This afternoon I will have my echogram done at the Arizona Heart Institute. Please say prayers that the results come back as normal. I am hoping to be squeezed in for an appointment to have my table tilt test on Tuesday afternoon at a hospital in Phoenix. I also get to see my primary care doctor on Tuesday morning for a checkup.

After this round of exams, I will be ready for the Ketamine procedure. I will let you all know how Monday and Tuesday go. Once again, thanks for the love, support and prayers. Everything you are doing helps!

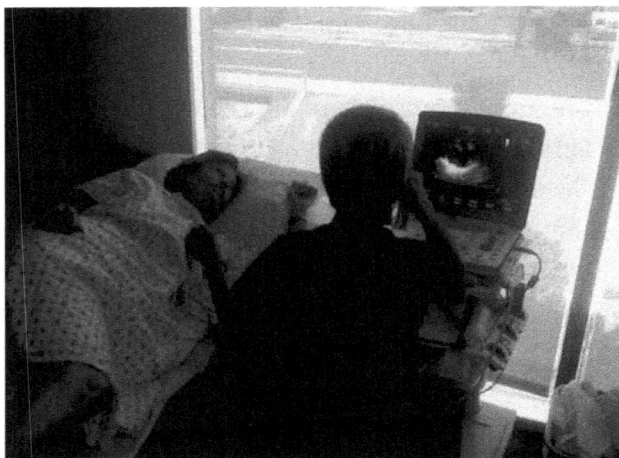

Barby having Heart Ultrasound

June 4, 2009

Yesterday was a miserable day. I tried taking Toradol, a non-narcotic pain medication, but within an hour I was vomiting and that continued into the night. I had a spike in my fever, which got up to 102.6 and, of course, had major pain. I did not get in for the table tilt test yet. I am trying again for next Tuesday. Apparently, there are not many places to go for this test. I will let you all know what it was like, hopefully soon.

As far as the echogram, the test went fine. The tech could not give me any results but she did not seem worried about anything she saw. I did not think that this test would hurt as bad as it did. She said the bone is so thick and to see the heart she had to press firm.

Well, when she was pressing between my ribs, it felt like she was trying to separate them! The exam lasted about

15 minutes and she did the pictures in color (showing blood flow), as well in black and white. I could see all four chambers of my heart on the screen. There were also three electrodes attached to me so they could monitor my heart rate, so I could hear my heart beating and it sounded normal to me. I am so ready for all of this to be done.

June 15, 2009

I received my results from my echogram today and they came back normal. I am still waiting for an opening at the hospital for the table tilt exam and hope to hear something by Wednesday. Then, I will be ready for the procedure and all I have to do is raise the remaining funds needed and wait. Yesterday, Ken and I met with a woman from the community who runs a foundation. Their mission is to support people from Arizona in times of need with their medical expenses. Wherever there is need or injustice, they can offer resources regardless of economic status or affiliation. They have offered to assist me in raising the rest of the personal medical funds I need for my Ketamine procedure.

June 25, 2009

I finally got my time and date scheduled for my table tilt exam (cardiac test). It is next Wednesday. I am very excited because this is my last test before Ketamine. *\o/*

July 18, 2009

I have had a rough few weeks but I did get my table tilt exam and a new EKG. The table tilt exam came back in the low - normal range, however the results of this EKG were the same as the original: abnormal. In spite of that, the cardiac doctor approved me for the Ketamine procedure. Now it is a waiting game.

The table tilt exam was different than I expected. They strap you to a table with three straps and then tilt the table up to a 70-degree angle. I was in that position for 40 minutes and I was in sheer pain the whole time. I got a little dizzy and nauseous, but stuck it out so that I could be cleared. My left arm had a blood pressure cuff, IV line and oxygen monitor. My blood pressure was so low that the machine only picked it up every two or three times it tried. Every time the blood pressure check was taken, the IV line would be cut off and blood would come back out the IV tube. By the time that the blood was back in and saline was flowing it was time for another blood pressure check. I do not think I got any IV fluid. Once the test is over, they bring the bed back down so it is parallel with the floor. For me, though, it felt like I was upside down. The feeling lasted about twenty minutes. The cardiac doctor did the repeat EKG, which came back abnormal as I said above. I will see the cardiac doctor in the next few weeks to discuss the exact problem with my heart and what we can do about it, if anything.

Reflex Sympathetic Dystrophy does affect your autonomic system, so to me it would seem that there would be an effect on the heart since it is an 'automatic' organ.

August 18, 2009

I finally got my heart test results and it turns out I have

cardiac ischemia. This is when the flow of oxygen-rich blood to the heart muscle is impeded, resulting in inadequate oxygenation of the heart. At the end of this month, I am undergoing a nuclear scan stress test. A nuclear stress test measures blood flow to your heart muscle at rest and during stress. During the test, a radioactive substance is injected into your bloodstream. This substance mixes with your blood and travels to your heart. A special scanner, which detects the radioactive material in your heart, creates images of your heart muscle. After that, I will find out what the cardiologist wants to do.

I also got a call from Dr. Schwartzman's nurse letting me know I could be called anytime between now and February 2010. I am excited because I am having some very rough days. Some days I only get through by prayers and hope. Just knowing that there can be an end to this is keeping me going.

X-Ray's and Blood Tests

In addition to the other testing, I have to get an x-ray of my chest to make sure my lungs are clear. This was an easy test. I was in and out in minutes and everything was normal.

The blood tests have to be done in thirty days or less from when you are heading into the hospital, so those will wait. They do the normal CBC testing, but also check other organ functions and if you have any viruses. I have not been able to have a nurse or doctor draw blood from me since 2007, so it will be interesting to see how they get what they need in these tests. Just getting an IV line in for a radio frequency ablation would be a fiasco. An anesthesiologist would put in the IV line and then my doctor would come in to do the procedure. He would have to manipulate the line in my arm, hand or elbow (where ever they put it) at that particular moment so I could be given the sedation medicine. Once I would fall asleep I am not sure how much longer it worked, but probably not long, seeing sometimes he had to hold it in place with his hand and it would stop when he let go. I cannot imagine that someone would be assigned to holding my IV line while he performs the procedure.

3

THE WAITING GAME

"All things come to him who waits- provided
he knows what he is waiting for."
Woodrow Wilson

Now it is time for the wait part of the 'hurry up and wait' life I live. I hurried up and got every test done. Crossed all my dots and dotted all my T's as I like to say. Now it is out of my hands. I am waiting for my bed and just have to be patient. In the meantime, I have no relief from the pain except heating pads, a dark, quiet bedroom and my faith that Jesus will bring me through this. Everything will be fine; I just have to make it a few more months. I can do it.

No Meds, No Treatments?

What is it like to stop all of your pain medications? It

can be very scary. I have many friends who this terrifies. I, on the other hand, was glad to get it out of my system. I am thinking clearer. Although I do have to say, Reflex Sympathetic Dystrophy does cause memory problems.

"What was that word I was looking for; my thought was just here, now it is gone. It is not going to come back".

The withdrawal can be the scariest part. I can say that for me it was about two weeks of withdrawal. I was on low doses, but had a very strong will. My will was to get Ketamine and get my life back. People who are on higher doses may have to go into a rehab program to detoxify. Others will just skip Ketamine because they are afraid to get off the narcotics and others will try to do the IV-Ketamine while on narcotics. Those of my friends who have done the latter did not have the results I did. They got either temporary relief, as in days or hours, or no relief. Neither were options for me. I was going to follow the protocol exactly, and I did. There is no need to question what is proven to work.

Lunch with Dr. Siwek

Dr Siwek, who is now my treating doctor in Arizona, found out about the foundation I am involved with and asked for a meeting to discuss how we can work together. Can you believe that during our meeting I got the call I had been waiting months for? I took the call and it was Carol from Dr. Schwartzman's office calling to tell me it was my turn.

I was so excited and Dr. Siwek, obviously being a pain doctor, wanted to find out more about the process and what I was going to be doing. We told him all about it and that I would be flying back and forth to Pennsylvania. I told him I was hoping that my pain doctor here in Arizona would do the follow up boosters, but that did not work out. Dr. Rubin did not even believe my Reflex Sympathetic Dystrophy had spread. In 2006, when I had asked him to look at my foot and leg, he did not. I truly mean, he did not look. I wanted a lower extremity nerve block for the pain and hopefully stop the progression, and instead, he insisted that I go to a podiatrist for testing. He believed, without looking, that I had plantar fasciitis. Well, I did what he asked and the podiatrist sided with me, giving me a diagnosis of Reflex Sympathetic Dystrophy in the lower extremity. I stopped bringing it up to Dr. Rubin at that point because I knew he was not going to listen.

Dr. Rubin was my pain doctor for nearly four years, but he was not interested in Ketamine and did not believe what it could do. I had stopped my radio frequency ablations for upper extremity Reflex Sympathetic Dystrophy in December 2008, so I was no longer seeing him by February 2009. We then started having complications with his billing department on bills from all the way back in 2007 and found his management staff to be very rude and disrespectful. Although I think Dr. Rubin is a good doctor, -he has to be: he diagnosed my Reflex Sympathetic Dystrophy in the first place- I know he has limited knowledge about the condition and he was not willing to look at emerging information in this field. He had been with me from the beginning of my diagnosis and it was sad to lose him as my doctor.

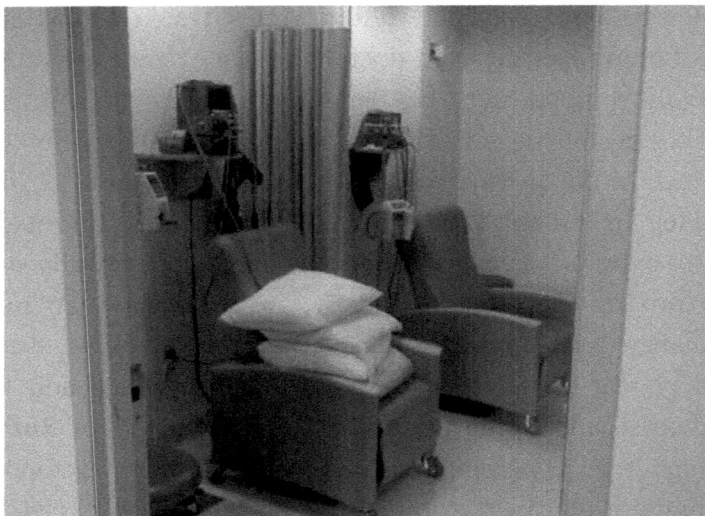

Picture from the infusion suite
at Drexel Neurological Institute

Sitting here in the restaurant right now, in this meeting with Dr. Siwek, I am happy I am in need of a pain doctor here in Arizona. While explaining the process of the boosters, Dr. Siwek said it was something he thought he could do for me. He wanted to help me, but I could tell he was still hesitant. We talked some more about the ease of the procedure. Basically, the infusion is an IV line, monitors attached to the patient and a reclining chair. While I was explaining what Dr. Schwartzman's booster room looked like, Ken realized that he had a picture. He brought it up on his phone and showed it to Dr. Siwek. Immediately, he said he had a similar room set up already. I asked him if he would be my Arizona pain doctor and provide me with the boosters I would need after the initial treatment. He said yes and that he would do my boosters!

Are you kidding me? This is the best news day I have had in years.   *\o/*

Getting the Call

October 21, 2009

Big news! I got the call today from Dr. Schwartzman's office. It is my turn to go for the Ketamine procedure. This will be the five to ten day inpatient version in Philadelphia, Pennsylvania performed at Drexel University Hospital. I will be in the intensive care unit for that entire time and will be secluded from visitors and outside influences such as my cell phone, internet, and texting. I think it will be harder on my family and friends than it will be on me. The bad news: I still need a significant amount of money to accomplish this. I am working hard to get this done, but I have a feeling of calmness and believe in my heart that it will all come together for me. I surprisingly do not have any anxiety about it at all, the procedure or the money.

I will get a call from Dr. Schwartzman's nurse in a few days to go over last minute procedures.

4

PORT AUTHORITY

*"I learned a long time ago that minor surgery is
when they do the operation on someone else, not you. "*
Bill Walton

I got a call from Lynn, Dr. Schwartzman's nurse. We
were going over all of the instructions and she told me to
get my blood testing done. I mentioned that I might have to
wait until I get to the hospital because they have not been
able to draw blood from me for a few years. She told me
she was going to speak with Dr. Schwartzman about it.
They have other patients who have similar issues. When
she called back a few days later, she said Dr. Schwartzman
looked at my case and suggested I get a PICC line or a
Portacatheter. It will make it better for blood draws, as well
as keeping a good line for the infusions. I looked into it a
little and decided on a Portacatheter because it could be in
for five years, takes a thousand pokes, is under the skin and

infection would be less of a risk. Those sound like great benefits to me.

Why Didn't I Ask Questions?

November 10, 2009

Tomorrow I am having a Portacatheter put in. This way during the infusion and the following boosters, I will not have to have an IV line or PICC line replaced every few days or months. The Portacatheter can stay in for a long period and is often used by cancer patients who are undergoing chemotherapy treatment. Getting an infusion therapy is the same process whether it is a chemo drug, IVIG, Lidocaine, Metamine or, Ketamine. It will take about seven days to heal from this procedure and then the plan is to send me off to Dr. Schwartzman to begin the Ketamine procedure. I will try to get some video of the procedure or at least some photos of the process.

November 11, 2009

Before they could take me into surgery, they had to draw blood. I thought that was funny, since I was there to get a Portacatheter because they could not get a regular blood draw. The nurse wanted to try, so I let her. After one try, she called over the head nurse. She looked and looked. She just knew she was going to be able to do it. Then they called over a doctor. He looked and looked. Finally, he told them to use an ultra sound machine to locate a vein that would work. They found one: deep inside of my elbow. I am glad I got it right before going into surgery, so when I woke up I would be out of it and would not care about the pain.

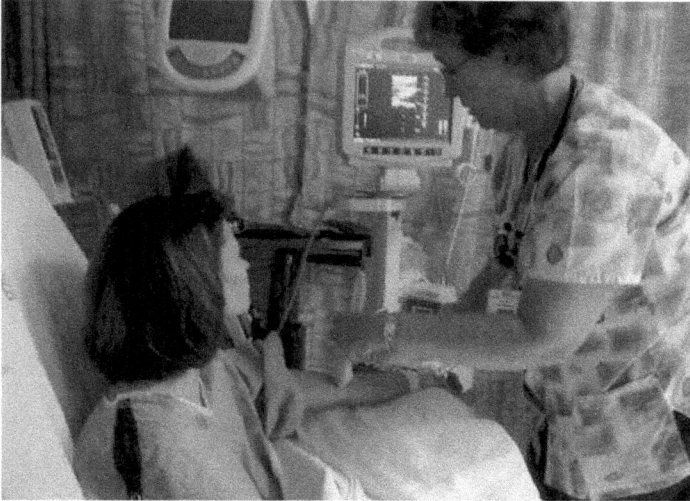

Nurse had to use ultrasound to
get a blood draw

The surgeon came into my curtained off area and asked me if I had any questions. I said no. I had had a PICC line in the past a few times and this was similar just on the inside. I did have anxiety about the procedure and was afraid to hear anymore. Now I wish I had asked questions. I should have asked questions. I was not prepared for the major surgery that it is. I did not know that the scars were going to be so big. Not that I am worried about how scars look; I have so many others, but I was not mentally prepared for the recovery. It was a scary, painful and uncomfortable time. In my speeches, I teach other patients to be fully informed for any medical issues they are going through, especially a surgery. I am sorry I did not follow my own advice going into this procedure.

November 20, 2009

I got my Portacatheter placed on November 11. It was much more invasive than I thought it would be. I have a scar on my neck and one on my chest. They still are not healed fully. On November 12, I began running a fever and headed back to hospital to make sure everything was okay. After that visit, it shows no infections were indicated on the test they performed.

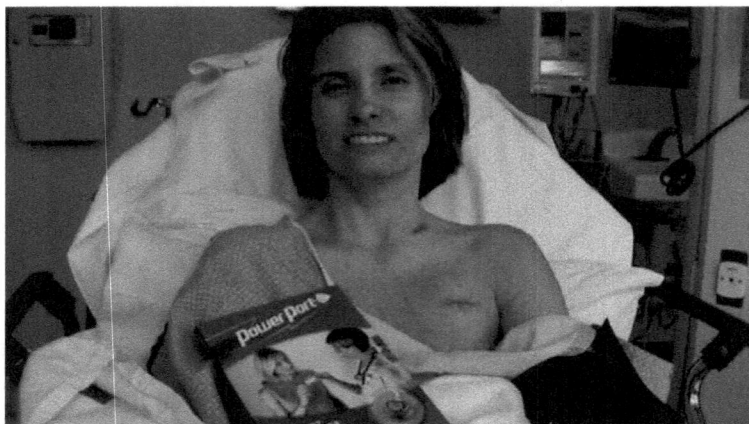

**Barby just out of surgery to
get her Portacath**

Nov. 18th was my birthday! I had to go to the hospital and have the port used to take blood. It was a great experience and it did not hurt. Shocking!

As they tried to get blood on the 12th, the nurse did not do it very well and it was very painful. The access line seemed to be stuck! It took my breath away when she finally yanked it out. The nurse on my birthday was great and I did not feel a thing. I am still having trouble sleeping and getting comfortable and used to having this port in me. I can feel it move especially as the swelling goes down! The nurse said the wound will be tightened back up and I will get used to it. I hope that happens soon.

The Trauma Is Almost Over

November 27, 2009

There are so many things I want to do after this Ketamine procedure. I cannot wait to start weight bearing physical therapy. My first goal is to walk to the mailbox and back without help or needing to take a break. My hope is that after the Ketamine procedure, I will be able to continue my fundraising to cover this life-changing procedure and the follow up booster treatments.

As far as a date to start the Ketamine procedure, I am told it will probably be about January 4, but could be as soon as December 7. The January date will allow me to work on getting the rest of the funding together, as it is a prepay procedure. Earlier in the book, I said that Medicare covers this procedure. Well I happen to be "lucky" in that I have a primary insurance due to my husband working. It is great in all situations except this one. Drexel Hospital said my primary insurance would not cover this procedure. Therefore, my secondary won't either, even though

Medicare would cover it if they were primary, I am facing a tough financial situation.

I will be heading out east this Friday, as there is a great chance the Ketamine could start on December 7. This would give me the time to raise or borrow the funds needed; also, just in case a patient cancels. Ken has taken on a second job and will be working weekends and some evenings to help with the financial aspects of this procedure.

My port scars are healing and it is becoming less sensitive. My neck scar is almost undetectable; the one on my chest is healing slower, but getting better. It is quite a weird feeling to have this under my skin and on top of my rib. The port sticks up off me so it is not too discrete, but the benefits are going to be great and I look forward to the ease of it as I go through this process.

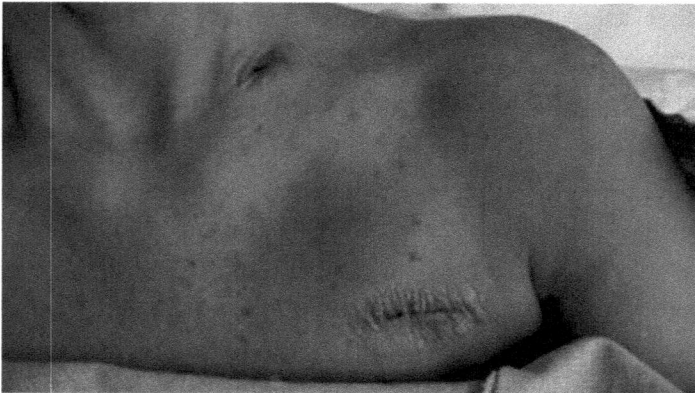

Scars from Portacatheter insertion

5

OFF I GO, AGAIN

"Wherever you go, no matter what the
weather, always bring your own sunshine."
Anthony J. D'Angelo, *The College Blue Book*

December 2, 2009

I leave Friday for Philadelphia. I am so excited!!!!!
\O/ Donations are still needed to offset the ongoing
medical expenses that will be incurred as I continue the
Ketamine protocol to ensure ongoing remission. For the
last seven years, I have had to deal with the daily
challenges of a debilitating disease. In basic terms, my
nerves (pain) are turned on and stuck that way. I feel like I
have been set on fire all the time. I am going to put the fire
out!

My doctors have tried all reasonable options. I have
undergone one painful, intrusive treatment after another,
many of which had side effects almost as bad as the

condition itself. My family and friends have had to watch, helplessly as I turned from an energetic, joyful cheerleader and coach to a disabled woman. However, there is one last hope.

What is my prognosis without the treatment? Because it took almost three years to diagnose my Reflex Sympathetic Dystrophy condition, it has made the disease extremely difficult to treat. Without this treatment, I will continue to deteriorate. There is always the possibility that if I get the infusion it may not work. I have done everything I can do to have a successful outcome. If, for some reason, it does not work, the pain, along with the progression of the disease and the side effects of the short-term treatments, will continue to take a heavy toll on my body and spirits. As time passes, I will become more and more disabled and need increasing amounts of care and medications. So this just has to work!

Following the procedure, I will receive boosters every few weeks to months, possibly in Pennsylvania. I hope that Dr. Siwek will still do the boosters when we are back in January. Seeing I will be the only patient he is doing this for, at least for the time being, it will be an interesting process. These booster treatments are obviously expensive, but they are vital, and an ongoing part of the infusion therapy.

December 4, 2009

I am about to take off for Pennsylvania. I am excited and hopeful. I have taken out loans for what I did not raise. Some people who promised donations or assistance did not come through, so I ended up taking out medical loans for the rest. While I am in the hospital, Ken will post an update each day. Please keep me in your prayers. So many people ask me about the actual process. I will explain as much as I know.

Where's Barby?

12/7/2009- It's GO time!

I say "our day" meaning Barby mostly, but also all the family and friends that have been here for support and I (Ken). We are all excited to hear and witness the progress. I will do my best to keep the updates posted.

After registration, there is no more contact with the patient. A phone number is given to the family to contact the nurses for updates each day. I spoke to a nurse around 10P.M. Barby had not yet reached her goal for medication and we were told that it takes about six hours to do so. Thus, a follow-up will take place in the morning.

12/8/09- Tuesday morning 10 A.M.

I reached Barby's nurse and was pleasantly informed that everything is going as planned. Barby's nurse, Colleen, told me that Barby is reporting her pain right now to be a zero out of ten, that she is doing very well, and that she is right where she needs to be at this time.

I had to ask again. Colleen repeated, "Barby's pain level is a zero. She is not in pain." I do not know how out of it she is and if she really knows what she is saying at this point. Thank you all for your prayers. Please keep them coming.

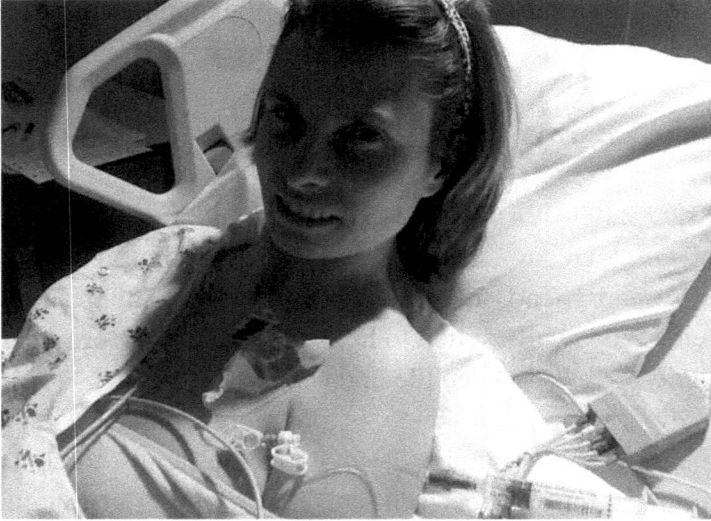

Just Arrived at Drexel University Hospital, getting hooked up and ready to start IV-Therapy

Family Feelings

12/9/2009- No pain is all gain

Barby had a pain level of zero last night, but this morning it went up while trying to eat a little food. Eating brought on nausea, which brought on the pain, so the nurse gave her some medicine to help both, and she is sleeping just fine now.

She is aware that we have been calling to find out how she is doing. She is aware of who she is and where she is at, just groggy and a little off, kind of like "she is drunk or drugged up" ...so the good news is that when she is asked about her pain levels, she is aware of how to respond if she is in pain. So, if she says she is in 0-pain level, we should think that she is telling us how she is really feeling.

- Barby's Sister

12/10/2009- Mobility!!!

Nurse Chris said, "She is reporting her pain to be at a level three but it will ebb and flow throughout the treatment. As she gains mobility there will come new limits that she will need to learn. The real test comes on day seven when she comes off the Ketamine to see if the pain will stay or go."

On a side note, he told me that Barby was watching *So You Think You Can Dance* and was educating him on different dance moves. GO BARBY ;) - Ken

2/11/2009 - Jumping for joy

The nurse said Barby is doing very well and is very comfortable where she is. She still has two days left to receive the Ketamine. The treatment protocol is for five full days with an additional day to titrate up, and another day to titrate down. She should be ready to go home on the 14th. I can't wait to see her. - Ken

12/12/2009- Great progress

Nurse Colleen said that she is very happy to see Barby's progress and that Barby is on cloud nine. She also said tomorrow is going to be the big test. Then, they will know how much the treatment helped her. So far, all signs are good and they do not see any complications.

12/13/2009- Get ready to go

Colleen said, "Barby remains pain free and ready to go home." She will titrate down tomorrow and be released tomorrow evening sometime. Barby has no pain when stretching her right arm anymore. Her skin color is back to normal. Sweating is gone and she is asking us to bring clothes and shoes that were normally uncomfortable and painful to wear for any length of time. Colleen said, "Barby is ready to go home, experience life on a new level and start living." I will see for myself tomorrow. I can't wait to pick her up. - Ken

12/14/2009- Picking up Barby

Barby's sister, her husband and I are driving to Philadelphia to get Barby out of the hospital. When we called the nurse to find out what time we would be there to get her, the nurse asked if we would like to speak with Barby. Oh, how excited we got.

Then Barby got on the phone. She said she did not know what the nurses had been telling us but her pain was not a zero, it was a three. She was very sad and we all got very worried. The rest of the drive we were very confused. Then her sister realized it was the bad weather actually. It was snowing. That could be the cause of the spike in pain, so we focused on that.

When we got there, Barby looked so good. She was so happy and looked great. Well, she looked good for someone who had been lying in a hospital bed for a week. We noticed her window shades were closed. She did not know what the weather was like all week. When we opened the windows, she was also thinking that the weather was the culprit of her rise in pain.

Barby was still out of it. But we didn't realize how much until later. She had her sister come over so she could tell her a secret. She had saved her Lorna Doone cookies. They are the best in the world she tells us. Her sister said those are not the best. They are only Girl Scout Trefoil cookies and they are crappy. Barby said "Oh" and looked sad for a moment. We brought up another subject and Barby sprung back to life. She forgot the cookies were even spoken about. We videotaped the whole pick up experience to put on YouTube. It was a very great day, happy time and full of joy! As Barby would say, "It is a Shake the Poms moment!" *\o/*

On the way home, we stopped at Outback Steak House to have a celebration dinner. – Ken

What an Experience

12/16/2009- Hey everyone, it works!!!

I am finally home. Actually, I got home on Sunday night but just coming out of my fog or "k-hole" as many people call it. My burning pain is gone, but I am having another ache. It feels like the deep bone pain, but it is not constant and occurs more when I am overworking. I slept most of the time I was there. They wake you up to eat and try to have you conscious when the doctors come to visit throughout the day, so they can do neurological evaluations to see your progress. Each patient, no matter your size, weight, or whatever, is titrated up to the maximum dose and then held there for five days, so the process takes longer than the five days. I did not know that going in to the hospital.

The first day, they take you up to the maximum dose over many hours. Once there, your five days start. After the five solid days, you come back down over many hours and then have to be observed for more hours before being released. My results were great from the start (at least that is what I remember). I don't remember much after the first night. Some of my accounts are from what was told to me after I was done.

Dr. Schwartzman was very excited to see the blanching gone. Yes, gone. My skin is white with no blanching; I need a tan. No sweating, no swelling and best of all, no burning! I did have a catheter in the entire week, except the first and last day. Now I am having some trouble with urinating and am taking some medication for a urinary tract infection.

I got a call today to set up my first set of boosters on Dec. 28 and 29th. It is a two-day process, which I found out today. So, typically, all of the patients follow the same schedule for boosters. My boosters will be: two weeks after the initial treatment, then again in two, then again at four weeks, and finally three months. Depending on how I am doing, we will do them as needed after that point.

Dr. Schwartzman said, "No PT, still!" He put it like this: They are bad nerves still. He has gotten them to be good, but they are looking for any reason to be bad again. So, I have to be very careful still. That is one of the reasons why it is *Remission* instead of a *Cure*. I also asked him if I could get off my Lamictal medication, which is a seizure medication also prescribed for burning nerve pain. He said no, that my body might perceive it as a trauma. My physical therapy will be learning to live everyday life. Finding my limits and trying activities will be more than enough for me to handle. I will continue to have limitations and much of what I lost with muscle and bone will not come back. I have to hold myself back. I thought I was going to be able to do whatever I wanted. This is definitely not the case. However, I am doing more than I have in seven years.

I am still very weak, and my legs are like jell-o, but I am so glad to go through these life challenges versus the burning pain 24 hours a day, seven days a week. It is worth it, and I suggest all RSD'ers try it.

6

WHEN CAN I
START LIFE

"It's no use going back to yesterday, because
I was a different person then."
Alice, *Alice in Wonderland*

I am doing well still. On Thursday, last week, Ken and I went with my little brother, his wife and my newest nephew to a holiday party thrown by his physical therapist. Many of the staff there had read my book and really wanted to meet me in person. With the Ketamine working so well, I was excited to show off. I was shaking hands, proud as could be at my progress. The doctors there were very interested to hear about the process and most had never heard of the IV-Ketamine procedures, so I hope I excited them enough to go and research how easy it is to administer it and how much it can help their patients. We need more doctors doing this Ketamine procedure.

While out, we started noticing that with little to no pain my vision was not doubled, I was walking more upright, as well as the no sweating, blanching, or vomiting. I started to get tired and worn out, and so did my nephew, so we headed back to my sister's house. It was so exciting for me to get out and actually enjoy the experience and meet people. It was also exciting for my family to see me doing so. They say I have a new glow and look of happiness that they have not seen for years. I am feeling very well. I just tire easily.

Dec. 21, 2009- Update. Trip to Dad's

I traveled for eight hours to my dad's house (which is normally a two hour drive at the most) last Friday night. The ride was so long because of the snowstorm that hit the east coast. By the time we got to my dad's house, the pain was an eight to ten level. The burning pain was back. The roads were slow going and there were accidents all over. The stress level was high and on top of that, the car I was in was very bouncy and every "ice rock" we hit reverberated through me. My seatbelt was going over my port (on the left part of my chest), and as the car bounced around, the seatbelt would lock up, causing me more pain.

I tried to sleep during the ride but was able to stay asleep for about an hour. The pain was so intense. I was nauseous from the pain and ready to cry as I thought the pain would never subside again. However, Saturday afternoon, it began to get better. I got to see my older brother and his family (wife and my two nephews) as we had Christmas dinner Saturday evening. I did not try hugging them until the end. Nevertheless, it went great and we did soft hugs before we left. I have only done air hugs up to now since the Reflex Sympathetic Dystrophy went full body and never got to hug them. It was one of my goals to hug my family members if the Ketamine worked. I got to fulfill my goal.

I rested Sunday and watched a couple of movies and the finale of *Survivor*. By then, my pain levels were going down.

It is now Monday morning and I am feeling good. Pain level is about a two in some areas, but most of me is at zero pain level.

We are going to head back to my sister's house in a couple of hours. I pray that it is only a two-hour drive and that the interstate is clear the whole way.

I Need A Boost

My first Ketamine booster is coming up on December 28th and 29th. Yes, two days. I found that out last week. The boosters are four hours each for two days. I will do this set in Philadelphia at Dr. Schwartzman's office and then hope to have my Arizona pain doctor, Dr. Siwek, take over the administration of the boosters from that point. I will have one due two weeks after I get home (mid January); one month after that (mid February), and then after three months (May). At that point, I will be reassessed.

As long as I stay in remission, I will not need to do the inpatient version again. However, any trauma can take me backwards and after the car ride to my dad's house I see how little the trauma has to be. As Dr. Schwartzman explained, my nerves are still 'bad nerves' that he got to behave, but they still want to be bad so I have to be careful not to give them a reason. If at any point, after the June procedure, I can start the process over if needed. If I come out of remission, and if I have the funding to do so, I would be happy and excited to do it again just to have the relief I have.

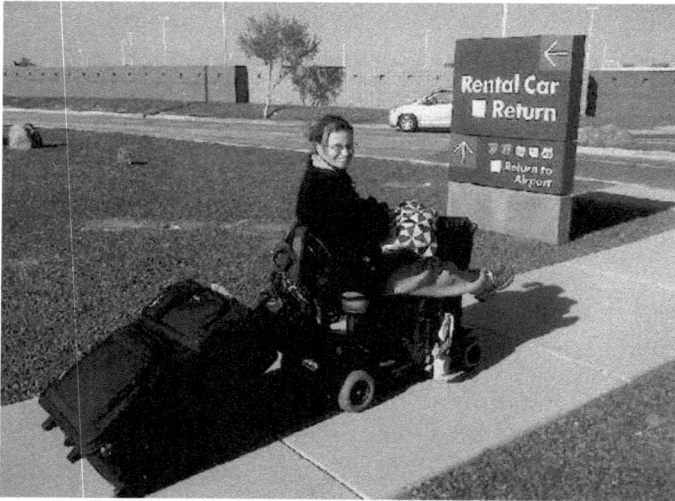

Back to AZ; last time on the scooter

Coming Home

Jan 5, 2010 - New Year's Update

Ok, I am back in Arizona and doing well. I got my boosters December 28th-29th, 2009 and I cannot remember much about it. Here is what I do remember:

I arrived at Dr. Schwartzman's infusion suite and signed in. That morning I could not remember if they said to take one or two Ativan, so I took two just to be safe. I remember the nurse called us all back and told us our assigned chairs, and then led us each into a room where our access lines, port line or regular IV line were inserted. That is the last thing I remember until December 31, 2009. Ken says I told him I was out of my body and that I felt like a bunch of blocks.

He adds that when trying to walk I looked like a bunch of blocks, which had to look funny. He said I was doing well until he got me to the hotel room and as he opened the door, I said I was going to throw up and went toward the trashcan. Well, I missed, and of course he had to clean up. ☹

The next day, he told the nurse what had happened and they gave me extra nausea medication so it did not happen again. After the infusion on the second day, Ken drove me back to Virginia.

We spent the next two days at my sister's house and then New Year's Eve with my brother, his wife and my nephew. We headed back to my sister's house at 2A.M. and took a short nap before leaving to the airport at 4A.M.

The flight home was a little bumpy in some places, but it was a straight five-hour flight to Arizona. We had no radio or movie on board, but we both took the opportunity to sleep.

Over the weekend, we went through our mail and were happy to see that we received more donations while back east. We also got a bill from Drexel Hospital for $104,599 as well as doctor, radiology, lab, pharmacy bills for another $10,000. Are you kidding me?

I spoke with the billing department today. We are working on getting some of it negotiated down and taken care of which will be nice, seeing that I had to take out a medical loan for most of the $18,000 I prepaid. It can take up to 45 days to get it all sorted out.

****

I am sure that we will be okay! God has brought us this far. I have to leave this bill in His hands. I have stayed at 85-100% pain free levels. The burning pain is practically gone. It has tried to sneak in here and there, but then I rest and wake up doing better, or wait for the bad weather to pass. I guess that is what the boosters do. They remind my nervous system to be "good," as well as making me remember Dr. Schwartzman's instructions to do no physical therapy. In the papers sent home with me, it was clear to "avoid injuries!"

We met other patients and their caregivers in Philadelphia at the booster treatments. It was great to exchange information and make some new friends who are going through the same thing. We have already heard from a few of them since arriving back home.

I am waiting to hear from my Arizona pain doctor about doing my next set of boosters here, instead of flying back to Pennsylvania. I do have dates set in Philadelphia, if needed, that I will use in mid January. I may be making another trip out east real soon. One good thing or bad thing, depending on how you look at it, is that on my trip out to PA, the airline messed up my scooter battery and it will cost more than two hundred and fifty dollars to fix. In place of the battery repair costs, they gave me a free roundtrip ticket so I can fly free on this next trip if needed. Moreover, I am not using my scooter anymore so I have time to get it fixed when we have the money. I don't have to stress about it too, at least, not yet.

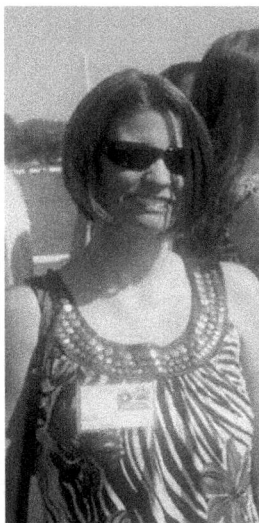

Barby at her 20 year HS reunion, 2010

Last night, I decided to walk to the mailbox. It is quite far from our house. By the time I got there and put the key in the box, I was already tired, and then I realized that... I had the wrong key. So I had to walk all the way back! Afterward, Ken and I drove to the box with the correct key, as I was hurting too bad to try the walk again. Oh well, I am learning my new limits. My mission is continued remission!

Come Look at This Girl

January 30, 2010

Hey all, I am doing well. Thank God. I got word this past week that my third in the set of four mandatory boosters will be on February 18 and 19th. This past Tuesday, I also went to see Dr. Hummel, my primary care doctor, who I spoke about in my first book. He was so shocked at how I was doing. I do not think he thought it was going to work. However, he was very happy for me! I did have blanching that day, but I do not know why. I also had a slight fever. The highest pain I have had since coming back to Arizona is a level four. That is nothing to complain about. I have not thrown up from pain since before the inpatient procedure in December. My dystonia was better. I had a glow of life that he had never seen and he was just shocked at how I was doing. He opened the exam room door and called the nurses and office staff. "Come look at Barby; I can't believe how she is doing," he said. They came in and were shocked as well. He and his staff never knew me before Reflex Sympathetic Dystrophy. They were now looking at the "after Ketamine Barby" and were so happy for me. I am a new person. Not the same person I was eight years ago, but who is the same person they were eight years ago. Dr. Hummel said he doesn't need to see me unless I have any issues that come up. No more regular doctor visits. Happy day! I wanted to go back to what I was before this all happened to me. I am going to work hard to do all of the things I am not able to do. However, I am finding that I have limits that I did not expect to face.

At the same time, I am doing some laundry and dishes. I have tried sweeping and that is still painful and difficult for me to do, so I stopped. I am putting dishes away, hanging clothes, and I even did some ironing. I am awake more and have energy that I didn't know I had, although there has been limits to that as well. Ken has to adjust to what I am now able to do; it has to be weird for him. He has never seen me do most of this before going through the IV-Ketamine because I simply was not able to do so.

Booster With Dr. Siwek

January 16, 2010 - Upcoming Booster

I got word earlier that Dr. Siwek's office (The Pain Center of Arizona) was able to get the Ketamine ordered to the apothecary. He will be doing my next set of IV-Ketamine boosters as a trial and if everything goes right, somewhere down the line, he will take other patients needing boosters. I am very excited. Thank you to Dr. Siwek and his staff (especially Michael Hardesty).

I got special messages from friends and followers through email, Facebook and Twitter. It makes me feel so loved, as well it lets me know that I am accomplishing my goals and touching other patients' lives. This one is from a Facebook friend, Shirley Stratton:

"I received your book yesterday (rather all 3 of them ~1 to my pain doc!), I am half way through and I am impressed. Very well done, especially for those that are newly diagnosed or even the very young. You relate to others very well Barby. I sense you have more than one calling/ mission yearning for you. Saying prayers for you always especially this coming week!"

- Shirley Stratton

Notes from her, and others like this one, make me so happy. I am excited that I am able to touch others who are going through the same things I am. I am glad to be an inspirational figure and a glimmer of hope for them. I truly believe that this is my purpose. I am a cheerleader and will forever be. People always would ask me how cheerleaders are happy and jumping around even when their team is losing. The answer: there is always a hope that we will come back. We can win! Until it is over, we can win!

We are working to get the crowd behind us and get a momentum going. I am glad I learned this skill and got to use it growing up. It is making me a better adult and better advocate for others. I think it is one reason I am able to get through everything I have had to endure. I always knew my purpose in life was to be a cheerleader; I just did not know in what capacity. I work my hardest now to keep hope to be an inspiration, raise awareness, and cheer on others going through the same things I am. I am an advocate for pain care and patients: the cheerleader of better life.

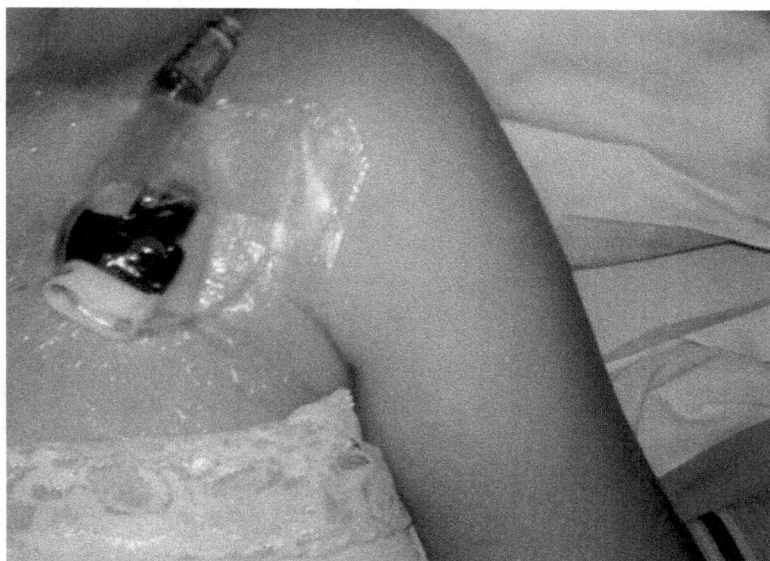

Getting hooked up for first booster in Arizona

I got a call last week from a special projects producer at a television station here in Arizona, who is going to be doing a segment on my pain doctor and me, detailing how Dr. Siwek is the first to do this procedure for RSD patients in Arizona, and how the IV infusion therapy worked for me. One day, I hope that more neuropathy patients can also get in on this treatment. Some other neuropathies can be treated with the IV-infusion therapy.

I have slowed down a bit on trying new activities. I have to pace myself and do not want to be injured and come out of remission any time soon. How about never? I am getting used to my port, although it does hurt. In addition, the weather changes still really affect me, and it's set to rain two days this coming week. ☹ On February 4, I will be speaking to a fibromyalgia support group on dealing with pain, staying positive, and how to be your best advocate.

February 17, 2010

I get my third set of boosters tomorrow. I am looking forward to it. I have not had the feeling that I "need" to get it, but I am still excited because I want to stay in remission. I am assuming everything will go like the last two times. Dr. Siwek will be performing the infusion here in Peoria, Arizona. He has a good set-up for his infusion suite. One of the things I have to do with the boosters here in Arizona is pick up my own Ketamine. The apothecary shop is holding my case of it and, as I go for an infusion, I pick up the vial for the upcoming booster. I think it is kind of funny, because the pharmacist always asks me if I would like a needle with my Ketamine. I would never try Ketamine at home by myself. I would only do it under supervision. With the side effects of hallucinations and anxiety, without the other medications involved in the process and having lower heart rate during the infusion, I am not comfortable doing it without healthcare professionals present.

The other difference is that Dr. Schwartzman has you take Ativan medication before you arrive. The Versed, Ketamine, anti-nauseous and Clonidine are given to you in your IV bag. With Dr. Siwek, he has me take the Ativan and Clonidine before I arrive. With the drive being over an hour, by the time I get to his office I am out of it and do not really remember or know what is going on, even before we start. Dr. Siwek mixes the Ketamine into the IV solution bag and then puts the Versed and anti-nauseous into a different access point in the IV line so I get it all at once up front, before the Ketamine starts.

In between the day of boosters, I am out of it. Remember, I am tiny; about 100 lbs. I have other friends who are 200+ lbs. We all get the same dose using Dr. Schwartzman's protocol. Some of them stay awake during the boosters, while I am out of it totally. I do wear a headset with music playing. As they start the Ketamine drip, I always listen to "Bubbly" by Colbie Caillat. It just gives me positive thoughts as I fall asleep. They also told me that during the infusions, if an earpiece falls out, I pout to get the nurses' attention so they can put it back in my ear for me.

My phone is my music player, so I have also texted random strings of letters to my husband and a friend while getting a booster infusion. It is funny because it looks like I am actually making words. I probably have something specific I am saying, but no one would know what I was talking about. After that, I totally get why they do not want you to connect with outside people, especially while in ICU. They say it is because they do not want you to be using your thinking processes. They want the Ketamine to do its job with the least stimuli possible for the best results. I totally understand that and I do see how important it is in the process. However, I am sure it would scare anyone who could not see you and make sure you are okay if they were getting random, non-coherent messages such as this.

March 1, 2010- Third Booster

I got my third set of boosters on February 18th-19th with Dr. Siwek. I got my access line put in on February 17, and the staff at the Scottsdale Healthcare Hospital Infusion Center (Virginia Piper Cancer Center) was very helpful. They actually remembered me from the access line removal the month before. However, I did not remember a thing from then as I had just finished the infusion with Dr. Siwek. Everything went great with the entire process this time!

The producer from AZTV Ch3 in Phoenix was interviewing Dr. Siwek and me at the start of the first day. The segment should air sometime soon. I am looking forward to seeing it, as I do not remember the taping. Once I find out when the TV interview will air, I will be sure to post it. In addition, I have been asked to do a radio interview this coming Tuesday (March 2) to air on CBS radio called "Sunday Sunrise" with Vicky Carmona. I am excited to be getting so much exposure.

Ken told me I did some funny things. I do not remember any of it, but wanted to share, as the stories are funny to me. First, in the car, on the way home, I was petting a horse. Ken hit a bump in the road and I said he killed the horse. Ken said he was sorry and I said okay and was fine after that, as if nothing had happened. I also asked him if he saw the little people. "Where?" he asked. "Here in the grass," as I was pointing to a "spot of grass" in the car. Then, when we got home, he pulled into the garage. Before he turned off the car, he says, "Okay, are you ready to go home?" I said, "Yes." He turned off the car and said,

"We're here." My response: "Boy, was that fast."

The next night after the booster on day two, he took me to a neighbor's house to watch a movie. I slept through the whole thing. However, at one point, the neighbor's dogs started fighting. I sat up and yelled at them to stop, and then fell right back to sleep. Now my neighbors have a funny story about me, too.

7

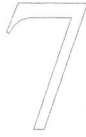

IT ALL STARTS AGAIN

"May God give you… for every storm a rainbow,
for every tear a smile, for every care a promise and a
blessing in each trial. For every problem life sends,
a faithful friend to share, for every sigh a sweet
song and an answer for each prayer."
Frédérick Jézégou

As I was saying earlier, weather changes suck. My pain goes up a couple of days before the storm gets here. The barometric pressure is what is actually affecting me the most instead of the storms. Either is bad, but before and after is worse than when the storm is directly over me.

April 26, 2010
I am doing a blogtalk.com radio interview with Trudy Thomas from "Living with Hope" tonight. I am really looking forward to being on the air, sharing my knowledge,

and advocating for patients. I cannot wait to share my story, tips and tell everyone about my book, *RSD in Me*!

Last week we had a few storms come through here in Arizona. In addition, a little over a week ago, I stepped on a bed rail and it punctured the bottom of my foot. All week I was feeling bad and need to do the IV-Ketamine booster soon. I was also having terrible headaches.

I decided to go to the doctor and get a tetanus shot. The doctor got me in on Saturday morning. I heard that this shot really hurts and was preparing. Well, the nurse used a pediatric needle and it felt smaller than a bug bite. I really did not feel it at all. Then they said that it would hurt worse the next day. So, I prepared for the worst. Well, I think that these people telling me to prepare do not know about pain. Yes, it was achy, but that is it. There was no pain compared to Reflex Sympathetic Dystrophy.

Well, I also found out that tetanus has the same neurological symptoms as Reflex Sympathetic Dystrophy; who would have known? It makes me think back and maybe last week I was not doing badly because of the storm, it may have been tetanus. I am feeling like I need to do a Ketamine booster soon; I am going to let my doctor know, so that I can possibly move it up from 20/21 to the 13/14 of May. I hope that will work with Dr. Siwek's schedule.

Who Put That There?

May 2, 2010
I have decided to get my next booster set early because

of the injury when I stepped on a bedrail a few weeks ago. The puncture in the bottom of my foot hurts, as well as burning, swelling, discoloring, etc. It has been bothering me quite a bit. I did end up getting a tetanus shot last weekend and did start to feel better overall after that, but still think it is a good idea to get it early. It will be two weeks early. I will be doing it here in Arizona with Dr. Siwek again. I will get my access line put into my port on Wednesday and then do the IV-Ketamine boosters Thursday and Friday and get the access line taken out Friday afternoon. I am expecting I won't remember anything once again until about Sunday. I am hoping all the pain (yes, I have had a little burning, since hurting my foot), neurological symptoms, and headaches will be gone again.

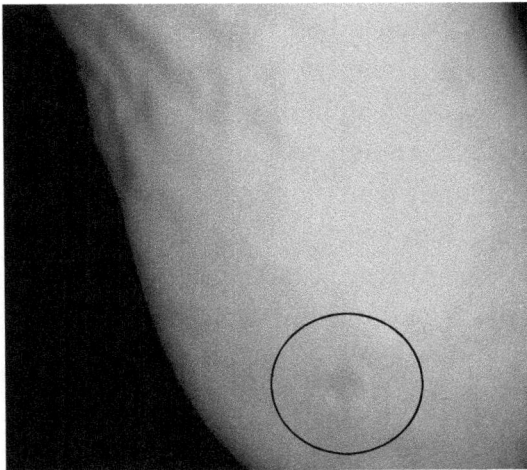

Barby's foot as it heals from the puncture wound

Ken and I did get tickets to go to American Idol again so later this month we plan to go the finale. It will be two weeks after my next booster so I should be feeling good when we go. I had so much fun last year while in pain, I am sure it will be even more fun being in remission.

May 20, 2010

I actually got my K-booster May 6-7th, which was sooner than I thought they were going to be able to do. Everything went great. I am now 85-90% pain free. I have to say 85% because storms still get me. Luckily, we have been having great weather, so I am doing very well. I have been focusing on the Power of Pain Foundation's events coming up. We just had two events in Virginia this past Monday and Tuesday, with over 138 in attendance raising awareness and advocacy for pain patients. I did not attend those, but am excited to hear that they were a success.

At the end of June, we are hosting an opening night showing of Twilight: Eclipse here in Chandler, Arizona as a fundraiser and awareness event for Reflex Sympathetic Dystrophy, chronic pain rights and advocacy in general.

Personally, Ken and I will be heading to Los Angeles for the finale of American Idol again this year. This time, I can do so much more while we are there. I am so looking forward to it. We leave next Tuesday and come back on Thursday.

I have come full circle. Just last year I was diagnosed with full body Reflex Sympathetic Dystrophy in Pennsylvania and then headed straight to the American Idol finale. I was not feeling good at all and the pain was sky high. One year later, I am on the other end of the spectrum. I got a new dress and going to get dressed up for first time since my wedding in 2007. I am going to have my hair and makeup done. I love my dress and hope we get good seats. We will not find out until we arrive. I will let everyone know how it goes.

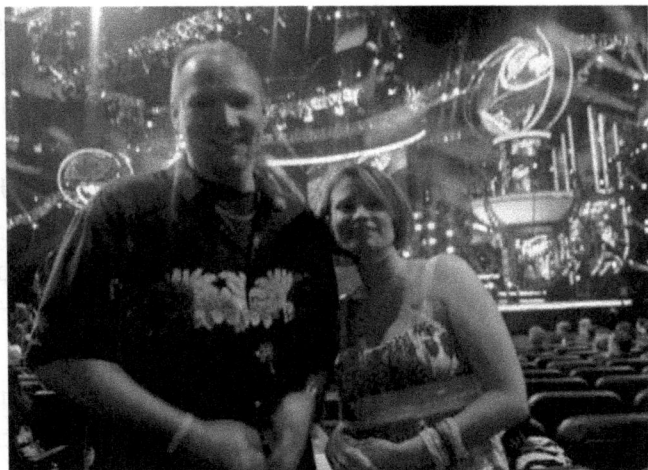

American Idol Finale 2010

American Idol turned out to be amazing this year. We were in row 11 on stage right. We were sitting where all of the former idols were seated. We were seats away from Scott MacIntyre, Jordan Sparks, David Archuleta, and the Brittenum Brothers (twins that were kicked off a few years ago after being arrested). Oh, they were in our hotel also. We were also on the same hotel room floor as Christina Aguilera. Ken saw her at the hotel before the show; we both saw her coming back afterwards. We did not get to speak with her, though. The red carpet was done differently this year and the fans were kept away with barriers, so we did not get any up-close interaction with special guests. There were a few in the lobby, but I was too worried about us having sneaked the camera into the facility that I was only focused on that. I am not good at breaking the rules.

I knew there was a chance that Paula Abdul, my heroine, was going to be there based on the tweet she had sent out earlier in the day. I wanted to be able to snap a picture of her, or her and me, if the opportunity arose. Unfortunately, it did not happen. I mean, her and me together in a picture. I did get pictures of her onstage. We also saw Janet Jackson, Bret Michaels, Christina Aguilera, all the former idols performing live and more. There were other performers as well as 'stars' sprinkled throughout floor seating in the audience. It was fabulous.

When we were walking out of the show, we were right with all of the former idols leaving. I really did not know what to say to them except Scott MacIntyre. He is from Arizona and was one of our favorites over the years so we stopped to let him know. He was with his beautiful fiancee. They were both gracious as can be. He told us about his upcoming show in Arizona in October and invited us to come. You know we will do everything we can to be there.

During the day, we asked around until we found out where the after party was going to be. When the show was over, we headed to the location. There was another restaurant across the street, so we stopped there to eat and wait for the after party to start. We could see the staff setting up but no one had arrived yet. However, by the time the food came, my body had given out on me. So instead of sticking around for Paula to arrive, we headed back to the hotel to go to bed. I tried my hardest to make it to meet Paula; I just could not do it physically. That was a letdown, but I know I tried my hardest. It is one more reminder that there are limitations, even in remission.

I am realizing how much I have taken on and it all seems to be coming at me very fast. I am so excited to be doing so well, I want to do everything I can. I just hope my body sticks all the activities out with me. In June, there will be many preparations for the movie night event. July, we will be doing a community corner event at the Arizona Diamondbacks game. This will help us prepare for September's event: Pain Awareness Day at the Park. September will be very busy. I will speak at an event in Virginia the second week and then head to Vegas for a week. I will be attending the American Academy of Pain Management's conference. This will be my 3rd year attending. After that is over, I will rush back to Arizona for "Pain Awareness Day at the Park" with the Power of Pain Foundation and Arizona's Diamondbacks the next day. Pain awareness month looks to be packed, and will be a great learning experience, while at the same time, it will be a total drain of my mind, body and spirit.

I hope I don't get hurt again. If I do, another IV-Ketamine booster here in Arizona with Dr. Siwek will be in order. Please say a prayer that it does not happen. I would love to have the next year with no incidences or major pain levels.

Lessons Over Coffee

I did not make it to September, let alone a year without incident. It is July and I burnt my hand. I could not get into the doctor right away for an IV-Ketamine booster so I was worried about the booster not being done in time for the procedure to work and would have to start over with the inpatient ICU version. I was trying to do more around the house and I decided to make Ken coffee each morning. I didn't realize that he had already made the coffee and rinsed the pot and put it back on the burner. When I picked up the pot to fill it with water, I saw something on the burner and swiped it. It was an instant burn. The pain had spread up my arm in hours and my body was burning by the next day.

I finally got my fifth IV-Ketamine booster (2nd day) July 26/27th and the burning pain went away again. We are still having some storms and monsoons, and there is now just an ache with some electric pains about a level two-three. I am happy to say I am doing well. I know I have to take it easy, not injure myself and keep stress low. I am doing my best.

September is pain awareness month and I am being asked to do more media and public awareness appearances. I love it, but I am also worried. I have two speeches, three radio interviews, possible TV interviews, pain conference, and pain awareness day at the park. I have not been involved in so much activity in years; I do not know how my body will react. I am going to take it one day at a time and hope for the best.

IT ALL STARTS AGAIN

All I Did Was Shake His Hand

September was excessively much and I am looking forward to October being low stress. However, I did not want to turn down any activities so I accepted events from September through December. I know it will be too much, but I will go until I drop, resting as much as I can.

Oct. 21, 2010

I have been very busy lately. I have pushed myself to my limits. It is not good for me and I know it, yet I keep pushing. I am almost ready for another IV-Ketamine booster. So much has happened in September and October. I still have so much more to go between now and the end of the year. Two weeks ago, we participated in the VCU pain conference with Dr. Hamza in Richmond for healthcare professionals. It went very well and there were a lot more doctors there than I thought would be interested in attending. I am happy to say that these attending participants actually came to the classes and asked good questions. They wanted to learn. I have been to other conferences where doctors skip out after they sign in and I have learned that it is difficult to get them to engage sometimes.

Today I am flying out to Virginia to speak at three events. Tomorrow I will be speaking at a conference for Virginia state workers, and then on Saturday, I am speaking at a Tame The Pain event.

The one that I am most excited about is on Monday. I am testifying with Col. Doug Strand, a retired air force veteran who has Reflex Sympathetic Dystrophy and has brought the issue of no disability rating for RSD military soldiers into the spotlight. He is getting some major press and I am so proud of him for leading this charge. I know how hard it is to do this work, especially when you are battling the daily challenges of Reflex Sympathetic Dystrophy. Luckily, for him, he has a very strong supportive wife who is right there by his side who cares just as passionately. We will be speaking to the Department Of Defense- Veterans Affairs Division. Can you believe the military does not have a rating for Reflex Sympathetic Dystrophy? A military doctor was the first to give a medical term to Reflex Sympathetic Dystrophy over one hundred and fifty years ago. Yet, they do not have a corresponding rating. They even have a rating for migraines at 50%. That is only one symptom we deal with as patients. If they were to give a rating for each symptom we endure, it would equal higher than 100%. I know the military doctors diagnose RSD, and even have some good treatment approaches for it. However, it only helps if the military member knows how to navigate the system for healthcare after they are diagnosed. I just think that is awful to do to our men and woman who put their lives on the line for us.

So, imagine this. I have been running myself ragged but this tops the cake. Here I am, it is Saturday morning and I am doing well. Just last night I said I feel like I will need a booster soon, so I am not feeling my best, but I am okay. I will be speaking at the Tame the Pain event in about an hour and a half. People are arriving to the event and I see a person who I met a few years ago at a Power of Pain Foundation event. This is the first time he has seen me since remission and I was excited to say, "hi" and shake his hand and show off at how well I am doing. I stuck my hand out and he crushed my hand. Mind you, I have a tiny hand and he is a big tall man with big hands, but what kind of person does a hand shake like that! It was the worst handshake I have ever experienced. The pain was intense. I grabbed his arm with my other hand and squeezed it, telling him to let me go, that he was hurting me. He laughed about it. I was in severe pain. It was obvious, and he did not even care. The woman standing next to me has Multiple Sclerosis. He did the same thing to her and she said her hand hurt as well. Nobody should shake anyone's hand like this. No matter whom they are dealing with: a pain patient or a healthy business associate. It is just uncalled for in any situation.

Now I am hurting bad: burning-hurting, Reflex Sympathetic Dystrophy burning. I go sit down in the back of the room. Within 15 minutes my entire arm was freezing cold. Dystonia, blanching, sweating was in overdrive. I was dizzy, nauseous and stressed. I still had to speak soon. One of the guy's colleagues came over to ask me something, I showed him what the 'hand shaker' did to me and he was just shocked. For the symptoms to come back so hardcore and so fast, it was a shock even to me. By the time I was to go up and speak, I was getting the dystonia symptoms back in my hand, arm, foot, and blanching up my right leg. I had trouble remembering my presentation and words. I had to hold on to the podium for fear of falling over in pain or from vertigo. As soon as I was done, I headed off to go rest. It was awful. I rested all day Sunday, but things did not get better.

****

Monday I had to go to Washington D.C to testify. It was great and the committee really listened. They asked questions and were interested in Ketamine. They seem to be moving towards giving Reflex Sympathetic Dystrophy its own rating for disability and they said they may ask us to come back again in the future. So, I think it was a successful day and look forward to the progress on this issue. I am flying back to Arizona in the morning, so I went back to my sister's house and rested up for the flight.

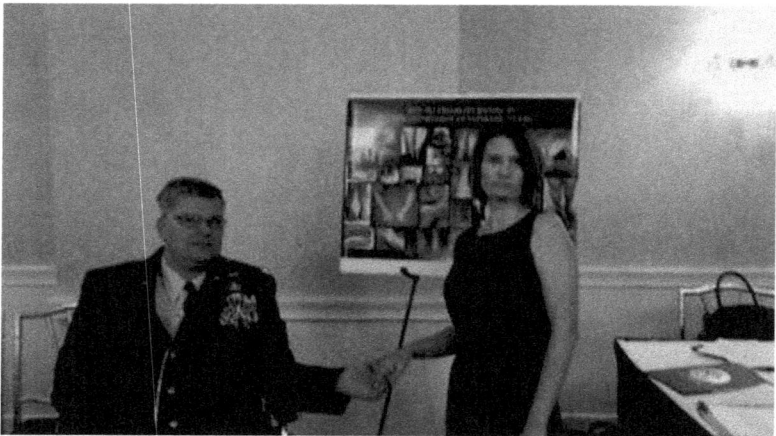

Barby Ingle & Col Douglas Strand, both of us are Reflex Sympathetic Dystrophy patients, before testifying at the Dept Of Defense- Veterans Affairs

When I was testifying, I got to sit down and read word for word off my notes so I had no trouble with my presentation and it all went off without a hitch. I have included my testimony from this committee meeting at the back of this book.

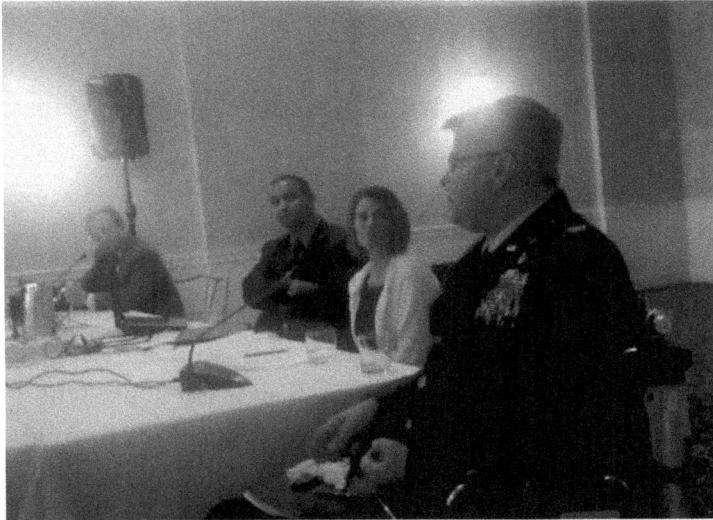

Barby Ingle & Col Douglas Strand, both of us are Reflex Sympathetic Dystrophy patients, testifying at the Dept Of Defense- Veterans Affairs

Oct. 28, 2010

For those of you wondering, I am in need of an IV-Ketamine booster after injuring my hand last Saturday. I am not on top of my game, ☹ but I am not dealing with a level ten pain level either, so I am doing better than a lot of other friends I know. I did get the discoloration, sweating, and dystonia and the burning pain is back. I will let you know how I am doing after my next IV-Ketamine booster.

At the end of October, I am going to the Scott MacIntyre concert. Then, we'll gear up for the November Power Over Pain presentation in Glendale, Arizona that I am presenting for the American Pain Foundation. I am glad I have a lot of time to rest for a couple of weeks, so I will be feeling okay for that event. I plan to get in for an IV-Ketamine booster as soon as I get back. I cannot believe what happened on this trip. It goes to show me, once again, I am not superwoman.

In December, I am speaking in San Francisco for a Pfizer conference, doing a pain management symposium in Kansas, and speaking at a Multiple Sclerosis support group event in Arizona. After that, I can crash, if I do not before then. The next thing planned after that is on April 1, 2011. The Power of Pain Foundation has teamed up with the Phoenix Coyotes for "Put Pain In The Penalty Box" night. I told you, I am busy and took on too much.

I know not to take on this much stuff in such a short period. I cannot do this to myself again. I don't think my events and projects are being completed as well as they could be, because I am not up for too much physically. The travel takes so much out of me still. The stress of events, even when I love what I am doing, and the chance of injury and coming out of "remission" is not worth the risk I am putting on myself.

8

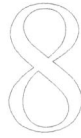

LIFE DOESN'T GO BACKWARDS

"Change is the law of life and those who look only to the past or present are certain to miss the future."
John F. Kennedy

As I moved through the last year, I tried to think about the future and what I wanted to do. It is simple: I want my future to be working, teaching and advocating, so others do not have my past. I am proud of all of my life accomplishments and look forward to this first year to learn my boundaries and set new expectations for the future.

This healthcare system process has taught me that everyone matters. However, the only thing you have control over is how you act and react to challenges. I did not see this before my chronic illness. I mean, I heard it, I said it, but I did not see it, know it or believe it. I am not saying that everyone should get anything they want even if they have not worked hard. In fact, even the most deserving do not always get what they want and some of the least deserving seem to get everything.

Knowing that I am responsible for myself and no matter who I have around to support me or bringing me down, in the end, there is just me. No matter how much you feel entitled to having someone take care of you, because of your illness or whatever other reasons you can think up, it doesn't mean that it is going to happen. For example, just because I am not feeling well I should not be mean or aggressive to someone else. In addition, if I make a choice that affects someone else, they have the right to decide how they deal with it. Just because I want someone to do something doesn't mean they have to or are going to help me. Every action has a reaction. It just may not be what you expect.

As a chronically ill person, I have to do what is best for me versus putting guilt on others to do things for me. It is not always the best choice to play the disabled card. At the same time, it is not fair to let yourself sit in pain when you can do something about the situation. Say you are at a dinner party at a family member's house. The host keeps their house cold. That is their right. You can ask them to turn the heat up, but they will not always comply. You have the right to bundle up or leave so that you are doing the best for yourself.

There is more than one side to every story. Just because something appears to be one way does not mean that it is actually what you perceive. For instance, when you have an invisible illness such as chronic pain, there is something that is wrong, but everything appears to be fine. People do not always know what to say, how to react, or how to help if they were to choose to do something for you. At this point, some patients will choose to say nothing, others will advocate for themselves. It is your choice as to how to react to the challenge. Know that those around you may create assumptions and treat you with behavior that you think is negative. If you just walk away, it may be easier on you now, but in the end, you deal with the stress anyway when resentments build up, patterns form and issues pile on top of issues.

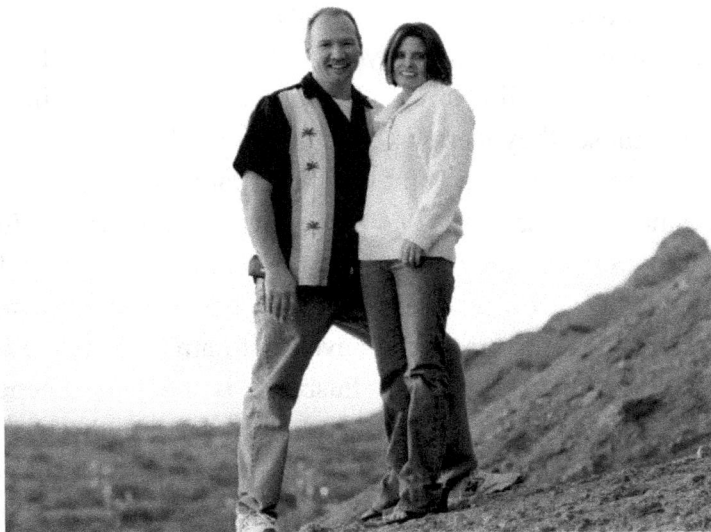

Barby and Ken 2011

If you have been the type not to "be your own best advocate," it is not too late to start. The good news is that it is not too late. Understand that people who have reacted to you in particular ways may be upset at the moment because change is hard. In the end, you will get better outcomes with the challenge you are overcoming. At the minimum, you will be better off physically and mentally with less negative issues to deal with. What happens when you do not take care of issues? You increase your pain, raise your stress, do not sleep well, and lower your immune system function.

Setting realistic goals

My experience has taught me that life goes on. It really does move with or without you. I consciously have chosen to go with what life brings. Some people are stuck in the same mindset they were when the chronic illness happened. For me, that is not the point of living. I am working to have the smartest today so I have the greatest tomorrow. Just because you are dealing with a chronic illness does not take your dignity, respect and living away. It just becomes different. I learned more than ever that I am responsible for myself and that even my husband is not my keeper. Caregivers can only do so much before they need a break, too. You cannot let others fault you, but also be careful not to put guilt on others. Everyone is different and handles the stress of chronic illness differently. Learning this and keeping it in mind has helped me in planning my future.

Cheering Again!

I got a call from a cheer company owner who will be hosting a regional competition here in Arizona in February. How did he know to call at this time? I have not had a call in six years to judge anything. I turned that one down, but with this one I was going to take on the challenge. He asked me to be the safety judge. That is what I am known for as a coach and instructor. I am all about safety and following rules.

This is a two-day event. I am a little worried about how my body will handle it, but I am ready to try. I love cheerleading and dance, and this could be my sign from God that I am supposed to get back into it.

Day 1

I check in with the competition director and told him how excited I am that I was asked to do this event. I told him and the other judges about what I had been through and how this was perfect timing. When the first team was done with their routine, I realized that this is not what I want to get back into. I still have the rest of today and all of tomorrow to judge. The music was thumping, action in every direction and I was having trouble concentrating on the routine. I did not enjoy any of them. My pain continued to rise throughout the event to a point that I probably missed some rule violations, but I was trying my best. Ken stayed with me the whole day. He was great. He went and got me water and lunch, and helped me relax during breaks.

When day one was over, I did not know if I could physically return the next day.

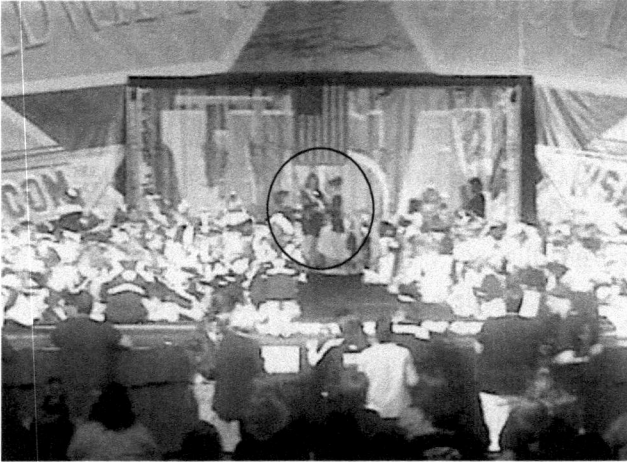

Barby passing out trophies after judging at the cheer competition all day

Day 2

Waking up this morning, I am in pain. The physical activity is getting to me, but so is the stress. Stress is not good for me. I want to do a good job, but know I am not necessarily the right person to be judging this event. I also know I will be leaving them in a bad position if I do not judge. So we head out for the hour drive. When I arrive, the building is full of excitement. Children are everywhere. Ken is protecting them from running into me. I took some Tylenol to try to get at least a little relief. It did help some, but by the end of the day, I was ready to go home. When I was done judging, I thought I would get my $200 for judging and be on my way. They spring on me that I will also be helping to hand out the awards. I am thinking, are they kidding? They were not. All of the staff goes up behind the stage and get directions. Trophies, banners and medals had to be handed out. I was hoping I would get to hand out the banner or medal each time out. I have to experience all three because of the way we rotated for each category of awards.

I started thinking and processing the whole event when it was all done, and we were on our way home. I realized this is not what I want to be doing and not what I should be doing. The participants deserve so much more from their judges. I am happy that I got to experience this one more time, but know that it is not the right thing for me anymore. As the owner of Cheertec and Dancetec and head coach of Washington State University's spirit program I had fulfilled my dreams. Who gets to do that? I did.

Looking back, I have been able to complete all of my dreams and life goals set at a young age. I was becoming complacent and not realizing how successful I had become. I was just moving through and looking past the greatness around me. I was not dancing every day, as my dad likes to say. Then I developed Reflex Sympathetic Dystrophy and it was taken away. I realized how much I lost and how far I fell. I went from the top of the world to food stamps and government assistance. It is time I make new dreams, goals, and aspirations. Of course, my body has to agree also. I will be working on a new list of life experiences to accomplish.

June 14, 2010

This is just a quick update to let everyone know that things are going well for me. Storms still get me, but I am good. This past Saturday we had a storm and I started to vomit from pain. It was a bad night. The storm left and I am doing better.

I found out today that one of my friends is in remission. It is a great day when I get a call that another person is in remission from the burning hell of Reflex Sympathetic Dystrophy. I am glad to be doing well and glad when I hear others are, too. It provides hope to those who are not yet where we are in the healthcare treatment process. I did get my port flushed last week. It was a new nurse, but she did a great job and I did not have any pain from it.

July 15, 2010

We are having many storms roll through the last few days. I am really feeling them and it sucks. I did burn my hand a few weeks ago. Instantly, I had burning in my hand, obviously. Then, it quickly spread to my arm and both legs. I have an IV-Ketamine booster scheduled for July 26th and 27th and, hopefully, it will not be too much time in-between the injury and getting the booster.

Monsoon season is approaching and I am glad to be getting the booster just before. Although, with these storms it feels like it is monsoon season already. This morning I could not get out of bed. Actually, just lying there was painful, too. I was cold, so I wanted to cover up, but then the sheets would hurt so much I tried to stick my legs out. In addition, the part of my back that was very sensitive to touch is back. No giving hugs for a while. I have vomited two times and remain nauseous. My double vision is back, too. It is suppose to be bad weather until Sunday... Yuck! I am looking forward to the booster.

Oct 3, 2010

I am doing well, still. I have been busy lately. I took on a bit too much, thinking I was going to be superwoman. It does not quite work that way. Unless I get hurt, the burning pain is gone 80-90% of the time. Other pains still creep in on me. If I get hurt, it all comes back: the burn, the sympathetic system dysfunctions, everything. I get very fatigued still, but overall, I am doing well. Ketamine has given me a good life and I do enjoy not having the constant burning pain. I wish this success for all RSD'ers!

Driving Again

I went in to see Dr. Hummel for a second visit since going into remission. This time it was for a standing order for port flushes and access lines when needed, so they do not have to contact him every month. He was happy to see even more progress since the first visit in January. While there, we were talking about how I have only gotten vertigo a couple of times since remission and that was when my pain had increased due to an injury or storm. He told me I am able to drive, but to stay on back roads and parking lots for now. I have not driven for years so it will be like learning all over again.

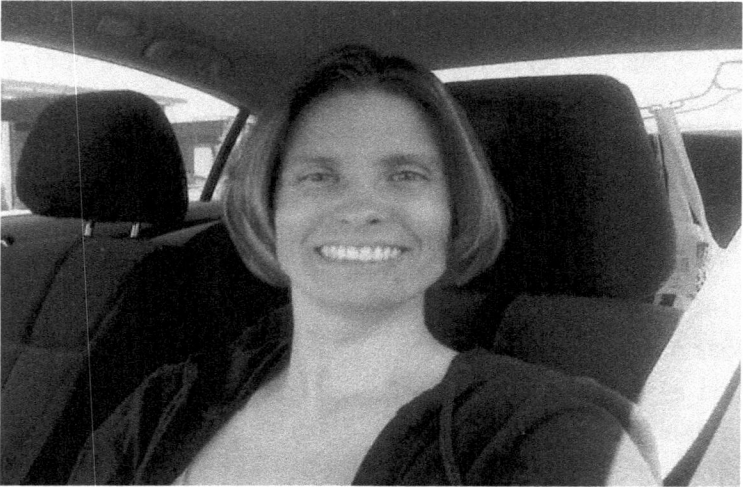

Barby driving for first time in 7 years

My first time driving I went around the block. I still have vision loss on the right side so I will have to get used to double-checking my right side before changing lanes and while backing up. I started going around the parking lot at the local school in the evenings. Then, I began driving to the store and back. Parking is still difficult for me. I try to park straight, but that doesn't seem to work out so well. It takes me a while and sometimes multiple tries just to get in and out of the garage. The parking spaces are sometimes tight. When I drive and there is no handicapped space available, I have to park where there is no car next to me, or let Ken park for me. I also drive the speed limit. I get to the speed I need and then put on cruise control so I do not have to keep a constant foot on the gas. I can also use the hand controls to speed up and slow down. My seatbelt goes across the left side shoulder, so I have to go around it or it is painfully rubbing on my port. The good thing about driving is I can go to the store, doctor, or post office without Ken. Getting some freedom back, even limited, is a great feeling.

Realizing Reflex Sympathetic Dystrophy is Forever, No Matter Remission

With all of the challenges this year, I know that remission does not mean the craziness of Reflex Sympathetic Dystrophy stops. It is okay that I will be dealing with this for life. It is hard. Do not get me wrong. It just is what it is and I have to deal with what I am presented with now. I also have to keep in mind how this moment's decision will influence my future. I have my great days, good days, and poor days. I know that I am not cured by any means. I also know that I am better off than I was a year ago. I am happy to have relief that so many millions of others are still waiting for. Keeping it all in perspective is what I have had to do. I have to look at the milestones from the past year and measure my success from where I was a year before that. I do know that remission is possible; it is just not what I expected.

But Now I Know The Relief of Symptoms

Are you kidding me? Before IV-Ketamine, I would say, "If I could just have one day with no pain it would be a dream." Now I have had many days with no burning pain. I worry about coming out of remission and having to deal with the burning pain everyday non-stop. I worry that the next booster is not going to work. I worry that I am not going to stay trauma-free and my body will revert back permanently. I have to not let it stop me from living. Even before Reflex Sympathetic Dystrophy, I had the attitude of facing my fears and even if I could not conquer it, I could say I did it. Within reason, that is how I am going to live now. I am looking forward and I am going to live to my fullest potential because I do not know when or if it will be here for the rest of my life. I will 'dance' every day.

Taking on the world

Now I am out and about town. I have been able to go to conferences and doctor appointments without Ken. I have done grocery shopping although manipulating the shopping cart is still difficult and I would not even try it on a bad weather day. When I do get out and do a take on the world activity, by the time I get home, I am tuckered and sometimes have some pains going on. Not normally the burning pain, but more like bone pain, joint pain, sharp pains, and electric pains. My heart races when I go too far or too fast, but I think that has something to do with the port as well as the RSD issue in this case.

I have been able to attend conferences, fly to speak at events around the country and see my family. The freedom is something I missed greatly. I enjoy all of it. I take it easy and keep stress off as much as possible. I travel light, and when alone, have some stranger help me with putting my carry-on bag up and down from the bin on the plane and going through security. They happily do it. I have learned to take breaks more often. Before remission, I was not even able to do activities on a regular basis so these issues were even more challenging. Now I know that there is a good chance that I will be fine. If I miss a plane because I cannot run to the next gate, it is okay. They put me on the next one. If a bag gets lost or I forget something, it is no big deal. I just let it go; I have to let it go. If I want to do activities that are more regular and last through them this is what I have to do, and so it is. Come what may, I will be okay.

Reasons to stay hopeful

I am hopeful because I have so many friends who are in remission and doing well. I have friends who are on waiting lists and I know they will soon join the "Ketamine club." I know that I am helping so many others. This process can be difficult to navigate and there is little instruction on preparing for the treatments and the life of remission. It is not exactly what I expected. I go with the flow and talk to other patients who have done it, and then pass on the knowledge of what happened for them and me to people just starting this process.

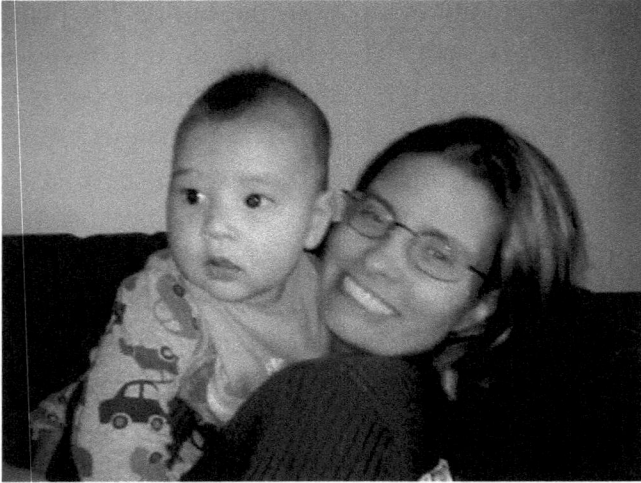

Barby holding her nephew for the first time

An IV infusion with Ketamine has not worked for all of my friends who have tried it, but it is high percentage in favor of working to some extent and long term. I know people who have done all three levels of the IV-infusions. Some of them have come out of remission, some have been doing well for years and a few it did not help or only helped for a short period. For the ones it did not help or only helped very short term they had one or both of the following. Either they stayed on their narcotics through the process and after, they did not get an initial treatment that was long enough to clear the receptors and have it stick, or both. I also wonder if the ones who do get relief would have better results in a more consistent climate. My friends back East and Midwest have four seasons and barometric pressure rising and falling is a lot more frequent than I have here in Arizona. It would be interesting to see if they come here after a treatment if the relief would be even greater. Can you imagine, all of the RSD'ers moving to the southwest states for more consistent weather?

For now, I am hopeful that I stay where I am with remission. Get boosters when I need and always have them work. There are no guarantees. Now that I experienced remission, I never want to be put back in the burning hell of full-blown Reflex Sympathetic Dystrophy and all the challenges I went through.

Nov. 10, 2010

Today I am going to get my access line put in so I can get my IV-K boosters tomorrow and Friday. I am ready and excited. I have needed a booster since October 23, 2010. I am happy to be getting it. I am also just getting over strep, so that was no fun. I am sure that had to do with my immune system being poor due to the pain and poor sleeping habits lately. My husband got it after me and was over it before me, so I do not think it would have been as bad if I was feeling better and experiencing less Reflex Sympathetic Dystrophy symptoms.

I did an interview at www.thepainchannel.tv last week that you might want to check out. They cover a large variety of topics related to pain issues each week. My episode was a great interview on Reflex Sympathetic Dystrophy, about being an advocate for yourself, the importance of keeping hope, communication with your healthcare providers, and using resources in your community to help you through your times of need.

Dec 11, 2010 - All I want for Christmas is a cure!

I have been in remission for a year and a few days now. How exciting. I cannot forget that I had three relapses. Just the smallest insult to the body can make all the difference in the world. I am so thankful for my doctors, friends, family, Ken and God. Without them, I would not be doing so well.

On Monday, I will be getting my last port flush of the year! Only four more years until I get this one replaced. I am not looking forward to that. They will put the next one in my right chest and alternate every five years until I do not need one anymore. Maybe in the next four years they will have a cure and we will not be doing IV-Ketamine.

January 6, 2011

It is a new year. I am still doing well. I have some good days, great days and bad days. Overall, 2010 was a good year with little mishaps. I did a lot of great advocacy work and in-person events. I enjoyed doing it all, but it was a bit much. I filmed two TV interviews on Monday and one aired live. I did not think that one went as well as the one that was pre-taped, but I only have great reviews for the live episode. I feel good about that. The second one airs in late January. Both of these interviews were on ABC's show *Smart Family*. I feel like it is a big accomplishment to get on an Alphabet Network channel. I just heard a few minutes ago that my friend who is doing IV-Ketamine for Reflex Sympathetic Dystrophy is responding well and good things are happening so I am excited to hear the great news. I have been saying lots of prayers for him.

9

SOCIAL BUTTERFLY

"Know thyself. A maxim is as pernicious as it is ugly. Whoever studies himself arrest his own development. A caterpillar who seeks to know himself would never become a butterfly."
Andre Gide

Since coming back to Arizona in January 2010, it seems I have taken off with activities. People keep coming to me and asking me to do media projects, speaking engagements and even go back to my cheerleading roots. I am ready to take it all on. I just do not know if my body will agree.

Media Darling

I was at an event in December 2010 and had a man introduce me to other attendees as a media darling for patient advocacy. How flattering is that. The goals I set at

101

the beginning of the year were to be a guest host of a show, be interviewed on an Alphabet channel, have three speaking events besides the ones for the Power of Pain Foundation, get 1,000 Facebook followers and get at least six interviews. I put this goal as my status on Facebook and one of my friends, who has known me since childhood, responded "Get a real goal; this is just a dream. It will never happen for you." I surpassed my goals and was recognized for it. I have done two TV interviews on the local news, two radio shows on CBS radio, co-hosted a show and been on as a guest for a blog talk radio show multiple times, quoted in newspaper articles, was a presenter for five other organizations, worked with state politicians to get better pain care policy, met with two producers from national shows and met hundreds of people across the country. I far surpassed my goal for Facebook friends. I am now at over 4,500. I know that I am reaching many people with my pain care messages for all types of conditions, not just Reflex Sympathetic Dystrophy.

I Got To Do It

This first year of remission, I was given opportunities to do so many different events and speaking engagements. I judged a cheerleading competition; testified at the Department of Defense- Veterans Affairs; spoke at Pfizer, Medtronic, American Pain Foundation proceedings and Power of Pain Foundation events around the country. I got to go to American Idol, to Burbank, California for a meeting with show producers, and was able to attend many other organizations events. I became part of the Arizona Alliance for Chronic Care and worked on getting legislation passed for Reflex Sympathetic Dystrophy, step therapy laws, and mandatory pain education classes for healthcare professionals in multiple states. I was in multiple media stories. I loved it all. I do know, however, I took on too much. I now know better for 2011 events.

I also had a whole bunch of friends who also got IV-Ketamine in 2010 and went into remission, or at least lowered their pain dramatically. I am so happy for them and will keep pushing our "Use Me, Infuse Me!" program so others can get this as well. I am looking forward to an even better 2011 with all my friends, family and supporters. Thank you all so much from the bottom of my heart.

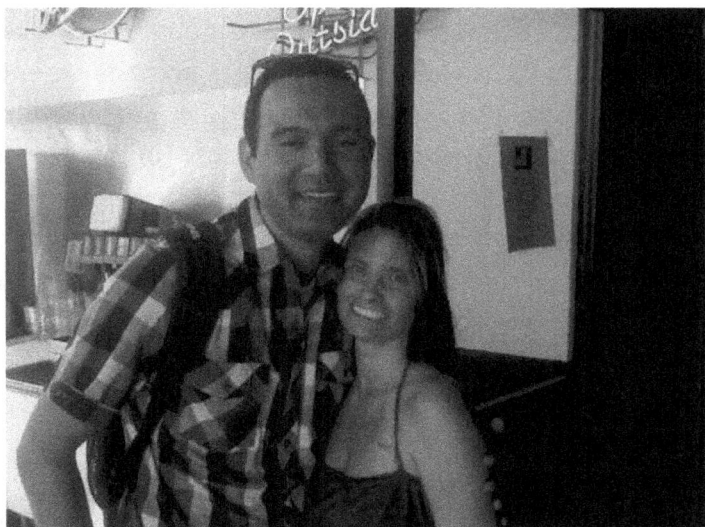

Barby And Kevin From Big Brother
At Casting Call To Get Ken On The Show

One of the personal things I did this year was meet some people that I have always wanted to. In the spring, Ken and I went to a casting for *Big Brother* TV show on CBS. Ken was applying to be on the show. One of the things that I learned was to do something so that you are remembered. It is hard to forget Ken and Barby, but just in case, I went through the interview process so that the producer would remember Ken better. She had asked him about me when he was in his interview, so I know that I had caught her attention. I was hoping that would pan out for Ken's benefit.

I talk to everyone no matter where I am; you could have probably guessed that easily. Kevin was a contestant on the show in 2009. He was there to mingle with the applicants and we got to talking. He told me multiple times that I should go through an interview. I don't know if he knew what the theme was going to be or he just liked my personality or story. I told him because of my Reflex Sympathetic Dystrophy and my port I was unable to perform the physical activities that are required. In the end his prodding got me to go get in line and try to get Ken chosen for the show. Ultimately, Ken was not chosen for the show, but I bet they both will remember us. Maybe a future episode will come up with a theme that is perfect for Ken and they will give us a call.

As I mentioned before, we were headed to the Scott MacIntyre show after attending the American Idol finale. The show was great and after the show we were able to spend time with Scott and his family. We told them about our foundation and we were surprised to hear during his show that he was a transplant recipient. He knew what pain was like; he connected to what we were saying because he has experienced chronic pain. At least it seemed he did. We asked Scott if he might be interested in singing the national anthem at the Diamondbacks game next September for Pain Awareness Day at the Park. I just got confirmation yesterday that it worked out and he will be representing the Power of Pain Foundation during the pregame activities and singing on our behalf. As I sit here writing today, news is developing. I have a feeling that there are even more good things to come in 2011 than I have had all last year. Things are going very good.

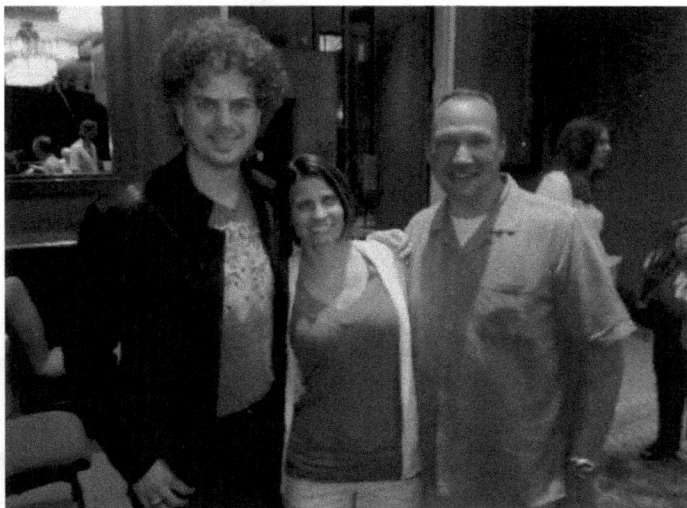

Barby, Ken and Scott Macintyre of American Idol fame after one of his concerts

I got a call from a producer in Burbank, California. They are casting for a new show that will begin airing in the winter. She was interested in having Ken and I come out to see if we were right for the show. This happened to be scheduled on the day of Scott's show. We flew there and back, and then went straight to the concert.

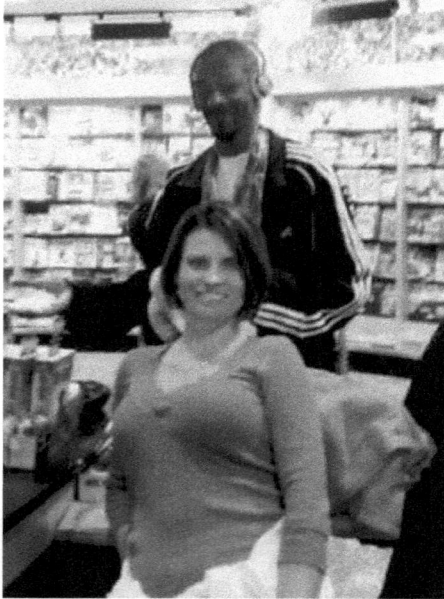

Barby and Snoop Dogg in Burbank while on a casting call trip to meet producers of a game show

Here is the crazy part. On our plane was the one and only Snoop Dogg. He was great. After we landed, he posed for a picture with me. It was fun meeting him. We were on a high from this experience. We still do not know if we are going to be on television for this show or not. It is hurry up and wait situation. I am used to that from cheerleading and visiting doctors. You rush to get to your appointment on time and then you may sit in the waiting room for an hour. A neat behind the scene fact that you would not necessarily know is just because you make it on a show taping does not mean they will play that episode. If they do not, then you do not actually win anything. Therefore, you had better be a really energetic, fun and memorable contestant.

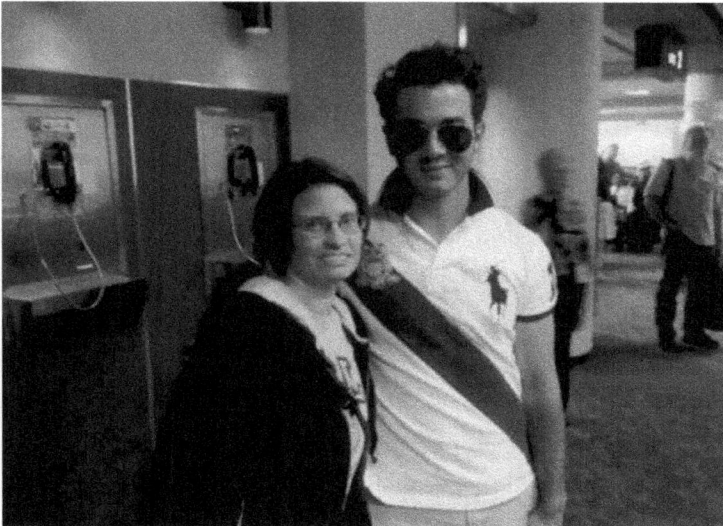

Barby & Kevin Jonas of the Jonas Brothers

So, out of order in time frame but biggest personal experience of all. God works in mysterious ways.

We were not scheduled for this flight. Our first plane had a mechanical issue and made us late, so our connecting flight and seat assignments had to be changed. We had been moved up from row twenty to row eight. The Jonas

Brothers were in row five. Row seven was empty and four bodyguard types took up row six. I hurried past the guards when the guys got up to go to the bathroom. I talked to Nick Jonas for a brief minute, but I had written him a note and attached three awareness bracelets. Nick is the one with diabetes. I gave him the note and bracelets and thanked him for his work for diabetes awareness. I told him about our foundation and that we work with diabetics with peripheral neuropathy and his work is helping so many people. The guards were getting restless, so I turned to one of them, said, "Ok, I am done. Thanks," and headed back to my seat.

After we landed, Ken had me go out right behind them while he got our bags, so that I may have an opportunity to get a picture with them. I was trying to find a way past the circle of guards that surround them, but their guards are good at blocking access and camera shots. It is like they practice or something.

They stopped to go to the bathroom, so here was our chance. Ken came up behind me and had happened to find Kevin Jonas's (the oldest one) wife's sunglasses on his way off the plane. At about that time, Kevin stopped us and said that the glasses belonged to his wife. We said that we knew and we had been trying to find him. One of his guards stepped out of the way so I could get in the inner circle and give them to Kevin. I asked him if I could get a picture with him. He said of course and we posed. Then I said, "I was the one on the plane who gave you guys the awareness bracelets. I know you will never wear them, but I know I thanked you for what you do for others." His response was, "You never know. We may wear them. Keep watching!"

It turned out that they were in town to do a live remote interview. One of the first things they did was give a shout out to diabetics who have pain. Wow, I was very excited. I know they did that because of me. How awesome.

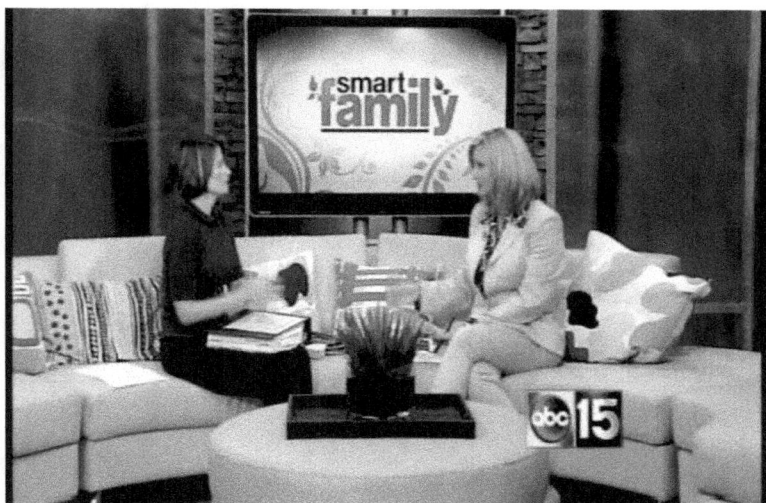

Barby Ingle and Connie Colla
on ABC's Smart Family, January 2011

10

WHY DOCTORS DON'T
DO WHAT WORKS

*"Never doubt that a small group of thoughtful,
concerned citizens can change the world. Indeed it
is the only thing that ever has."*
Margaret Mead

I know firsthand that IV-infusion therapy can work. Not just IV-Ketamine, but IV-IVIG and IV-lidocaine as well. It is a non-invasive treatment option. In the case of IVIG, it is very expensive to make, so insurance companies fight it a lot and this discourages doctors to offer it. IV-lidocaine offers some relief but is short lasting. In the case of IV-Ketamine, it is an inexpensive drug and insurance companies are covering it. Infusion therapy is being performed for patients with all kinds of neuropathy conditions and it helps many recipients. It is just hard to find a doctor who will perform infusions for anything more than IV-chemotherapy for cancer patients.

What I have run into all year is resistance from doctors. Some are doctors who I know very well, which sadden me. I started asking around for names of doctors who are performing the boosters or inpatient versions. What I found was that the list was very small.

I started asking questions to doctors specifically. I did not do this as 'patient Barby', but as director of the Power of Pain Foundation. I have my own personal story and many friends who have gone into remission from these types of therapies. Some of these doctors have seen me over the past few years. They cannot believe their eyes when they see me now. Yet they still give reasons and obstacles for not wanting to offer these treatments.

Financial

Doctors tell me there is just no money in it. They can put a spinal cord stimulator into a patient for $60,000 - $100,000, or they can do an outpatient IV-infusion therapy for about $1,000. Both take about four hours to do per patient but there are thousands of dollars that the doctors are not collecting. Technically, with an IV-infusion patient on Ketamine, you have a set number of boosters and then it is as needed. If you are active like me, your doctors will be doing more boosters. Nevertheless, many patients are not as active as I am and they do not take the chances. Therefore, they do not create new trauma as often, and subsequently, do not need treatments as regularly. So not only are doctors missing out from the start with finances, it is all the way through the patient's care.

From the other side, I see that doctors are underpaid. They are getting cutbacks from insurance companies and on treatment reimbursements with Medicare. Malpractice insurance rates are very high. Doctors also have thousands of dollars in student loans and they work for someone, making less than they would on their own. On the other hand, they may own the practice and make less because of overhead with the location and staffing. As a former business owner, I see the valid points the doctors are making. As a patient, I wish I could fix these reasons so that more patients could be helped. I am sorry to say I do not have a fix for this issue.

Insurance Companies' Hassles

Insurance companies give the doctors who do perform IV-Ketamine a hassle. More so a few years ago, but even today, some still get problems. Doctors who looked into doing these a few years ago decided not to offer the procedure or to do it on a cash basis only. I have found that insurance companies are covering it, although some of my friends have had to file appeals. In the end, my insurance company did indeed pay for most of my inpatient treatment; as well they are now paying for my outpatient treatments. I had to file the paperwork instead of the hospital, but ran into no issues on the portion they paid the hospital and did not file any appeals.

The FDA approved Ketamine for a specific route of administration (IV), dosage range, and including general anesthesia to treat breakthrough pain regardless of the underlying illness state diagnosis on February 19, 1970.[4],[5] As Reflex Sympathetic Dystrophy is a disease condition that involves breakthrough pain, this in effect is saying the FDA has approved Ketamine usage for treatment in Reflex Sympathetic Dystrophy.

Anesthesiologists have been using Ketamine to treat breakthrough pain in many clinical applications. It is used on burn victims, as a bronchodilator, and as anesthetic for children. Patients with multiple conditions are covered in these uses: people with pain, asthma, surgical procedures, burn victims and more. It is used on people of all ages.

Scheduling Issues

Many doctors have very small offices. Even at pain management and surgical facilities, the patient takes up a spot in the recovery room or infusion room for half a day. That becomes prohibitive for doctors to deal with because it cuts down the number of patients they can treat as well as amount of funding they can make.

To Choose to Learn Something New or Not

In medical school, doctors have to choose a specialty

---

[4] Janice Arenofsky, Ketamine Isn't Just for Pets and Ravers Anymore; People Living in Extreme Pain Are Trying It as a Remedy, Alter Net, September 28, 2009
[5] Federal Drug Administration, Approval History of Ketalar, Active Ingredient(s) Ketamine Hydrochloride, FDA Application number: NDA016812, February 19, 1970

area of study. They get general studies, but it is a little info on this, a little info on that. Unless a doctor is interested in studying the area that includes your condition, he or she may not even hear of it or be able to spot it or treat you for it. Even if they study the category your condition falls under, it still does not mean they will get any more than zero to four hours in all of their training on your condition. For instance, I know neurologists who are great, but they choose to concentrate on multiple sclerosis. When I have asked them about Reflex Sympathetic Dystrophy, they do not know about it or have any information. I end up teaching them. I hope that gives them a reason to go look it up, because they could help other patients they run across. Another example is that there are many surgeons. Some surgeons do heart work, others do joint and ligament repairs, etc. I have heard from doctors that they do not have time to learn a new protocol, even when they are standing there at a conference where they could easily get the needed information.

Looking at it from the other side, doctors do have little time for treating patients, and they have required continuing education hours that they also have to fit in. Some tend to stick to classes that reflect their area of interest. So they are not getting a wide variety of knowledge that, as patients, we tend to believe occurs. I learned the hard way doctors are not created equal. It may just come down to them knowing of the condition, but it is not their specialty, so they do not invest in it.

Have To Pay a Certified Nurse to Be There the Entire Time

When you have the IV-Ketamine infusions, a certified nurse needs to be present the entire time. It is different from when nurses can come in and out of patient rooms; this nurse has to monitor you the entire time. The treating doctor is present, but can be doing other things. Taking one staff member away for one or a few patients at a time for four hours a day increases a doctor's overhead expenses. Most doctors could not survive on this type of set up. They need to see more patients; therefore they need more assistant staff members.

Takes Up Space in Their Recovery Rooms

Not only are you taking vital staff away from other patients, you are using space. If you are taking up a chair in the recovery room at a doctor's facility for hours, the doctor is unable to fill that chair with other paying patients. Not just paying patients, but patients who also need help, just as much as you do.

Only Pay Attention to Studies and They Have Not Been Exposed To Studies On The Subject

Some doctors have tried to argue that there are no studies showing effectiveness of IV-Ketamine treatments. There are many studies that have been done all over the world. There were also over 300 articles I found while researching for this section of the book. These were printed in medical pain journals. I am sure there are more, but I figured that there was enough evidence for me that I did not need to look further.

Two studies that were done demonstrate the long-term benefits of this treatment. One of the studies was performed in the Netherlands; the other was right here in the United States. Both studies show that IV-Ketamine produces effective and long-term pain relief of Reflex Sympathetic Dystrophy.[6,7] The studies also used a control group, meaning some of the recipients got a placebo and others got the actual Ketamine. The studies also demonstrated that higher doses and duration plays an important part in how well the treatment works.

I have heard another argument being tossed around is no double-blind studies have been done on coma treatments so the FDA will not approve this level of treatment. Recently, I have heard of an IV-Ketamine Coma study being done in New York. I don't have any further information on how it is being conducted. The same standard should apply to spinal cord stimulators in my opinion. Insurance companies with a lot less hassle already cover SCS. It seems to make sense that the FDA would want to protect us. However, in both situations, it would be unethical to perform a double-

---

[6] Marnix J. Sigtermansa, Jacobus J. van Hiltenb, Martin C.R. Bauera, M. Sesmu Arbousc, Johan Marinusb, Elise Y. Sartona, Albert Dahana, Ketamine produces effective and long-term pain relief in patients with Complex Regional Pain Syndrome Type 1, PAIN, Published in the October 2009 issue (Vol. 145, Issue 3, Pages 271-272)

[7] Robert J. Schwartzman, MD; Guillermo M. Alexander, Ph.D.; John R. Grothusen, PhD; Terry Paylor RN; Erin Reichenberger MS; Marielle Perreault BS, Outpatient intravenous Ketamine for the treatment of complex regional pain syndrome: a double-blind placebo controlled study, Drexel University College of Medicine, Volume 147, Issue 1, Pages 107-115 (15 December 2009)

blind study. With the Ketamine, studies showing such promise as much as 80% success rate with inpatient and outpatient protocols, the coma treatment may not even be a risk that most would have to take. I actually cannot think of a way to do a double blind study with a SCS. With SCS, the patient has follow up surgeries, complications, battery replacements, and infections, all requiring future care. For me, the risk of spread, with the added trauma of surgery to implant the device, is cause enough to stop and evaluate. Do no harm is what doctors learn in school. As a patient, I want the least invasive treatment before surgery of any kind. It just makes sense to me.

When armed with this knowledge, it will be easier for patients to get insurance companies to cover these therapies. In turn, it will resolve one major issue doctors are dealing with when deciding to offer this treatment. I pray that it becomes widespread as an option. I remember back in 2007, I was at a conference where Dr. Schwartzman was speaking and he said, "It will soon be the standard treatment for RSD/CRPS patients."

The Good Guys

I have to say, over the last three years, I have seen more coverage of Reflex Sympathetic Dystrophy and Ketamine as a treatment option in particular. I truly believe that we are moving in the right direction. As information spreads and medical knowledge is brought to light at medical conferences, we will see a great improvement.

I am not saying that IV-Ketamine is the only form of treatment that should be approached. A multi-disciplinary approach is the best way to overcome the challenges.

Oct. 28, 2010

Today I have to tape my story for an upcoming episode for the Pain Channel. I just want to say how great this doctor is for me and I like that he uses a multidisciplinary approach with his patients. Dr. Siwek is doing my IV-K boosters and set up a program for other patients. The Pain Center offers a wide variety of treatment modalities, and they have many locations around the Phoenix Arizona area. The doctors there know that each patient is different and, therefore, must have their own assessment. IV-Ketamine is not appropriate for everyone and that is a determination for a doctor to make for his or her patient. As I documented in earlier chapters, many tests should be performed before you begin IV-Ketamine therapies. You can learn more about the Pain Channel at www.thepainchannel.tv; they cover a wide variety of topics.

Some Doctors Do Listen!

As I finish my book tonight, I got the perfect example of how some doctors get it. It takes time and work. It takes advocating for yourself, but it can be done.

I got great news once again today. I like the days when I get good news stories. A friend I have been trying to help was in tremendous pain and away from her family. Her mother called her regular doctor and left messages. They had no return call, so this young woman heads to the emergency room all by herself. Her mother's instructions were not to leave until they do something! When she arrives at the hospital she draws "a lucky card and gets an emergency room doctor who remembers her from a prior visit and likes her." The doctor actually calls the mother and asks what to do. She told him the only thing she thought that would help is #1 Admit her and #2, Ketamine or Metamine infusion therapy. Strategically, her mom offered Metamine as an option because this is the hospital that told her they use Metamine but not Ketamine during her daughters last visit. The resident calls her mom at 10 P.M. to go over her daughter's medical history and the resident mentions that she has worked with Ketamine before, but she will need to talk to the attending doctor in morning.

The next day, the attending doctor came in and she is one that gave this young woman some problems during her last visit. The attending doctor starts kind of "barking at the patient." So this patient tells her, "I don't appreciate you being so rude. I am 19, alone and on my own, in pain, and I do not want to be talked to like that."

The attending doctor actually stopped and listened with tears in her eyes. She told the patient that she was sorry and if it ever happened again she could call her on it, even in a room full of people. The patient said she would never do that in front of people, so the attending doctor gave her a code word to use if it ever happened. The doctor sat down and listened to what the patient's thoughts were.

It turned out that in the past six months the doctor has been doing outpatient Ketamine on another patient following Dr. Schwartzman's protocol. The doctor went up to the ICU unit and booked a bed in the ICU. She is right now getting her 5-day inpatient IV-Ketamine infusion. She is the first person in this hospital. This hospital is using Dr. Schwartzman's protocol and the outcome looks bright. This shows me that there is a way and doctors just have to listen and help. I really am proud of this young woman. She did a great job being the chief of staff of her medical team; that is for sure! Her story puts a smile on my face. Understand that this attending doctor was from the practice the patient went to last year, but left. All they offered her was a SCS. The young woman said back then that she would like to come back to them "if they would promise to stop pushing it." How great is that! A year later the doctor is seeing things our way.

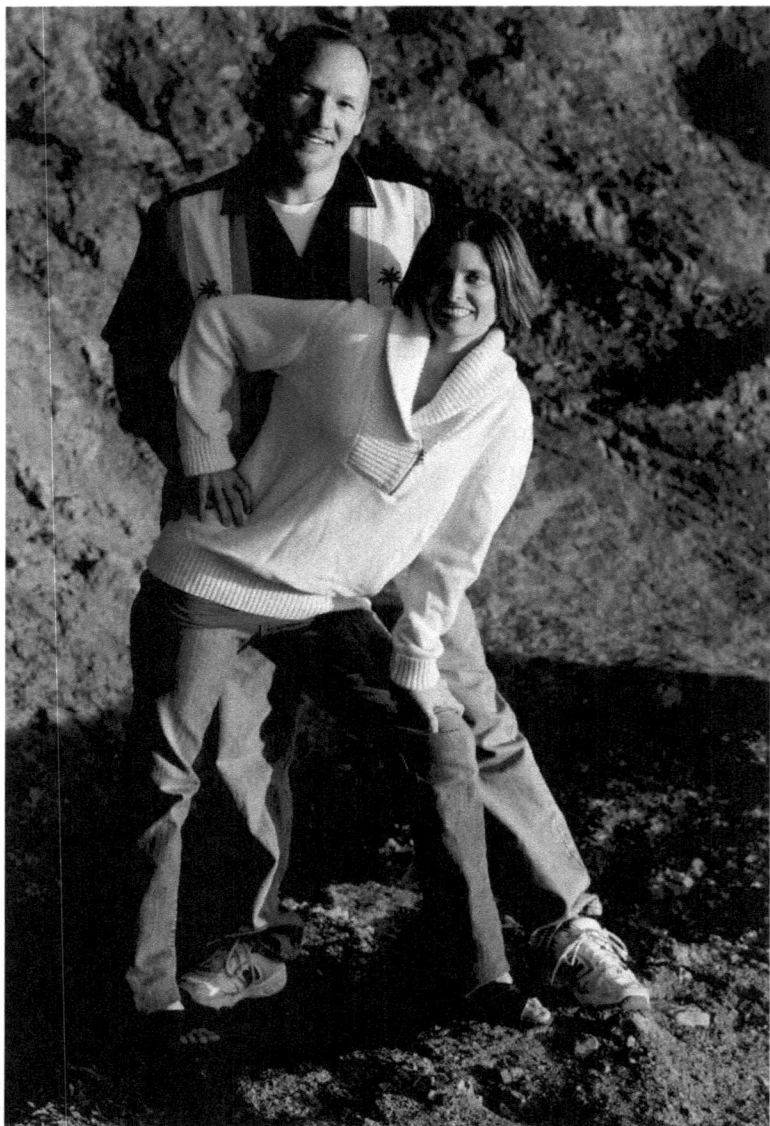

Barby Ingle and her husband Ken

The following is a partial transcript of my testimony to the Congressional Committee by Barby Ingle on RSD.

October 25th, 2010

MS. INGLE: My name is Barby Ingle, and I'm a bestselling author, patient, and educational presenter for RSD and other chronic pain issues. I serve as Director of the Power of Pain Foundation, which is a national not-for-profit charity assisting neuropathy pain patients. The Power of Pain Foundation's mission is to raise awareness and provide direct support for chronic pain patients, specifically those with neuropathy including RSD.

Because of a lack of understanding in the medical profession, I have undergone seven major surgeries, five pneumothorax, including a full lung collapse, and over 40 other medical procedures requiring twilight anesthesia in an eight-year period.

I have endured major complications from treatments and medications. It took almost three years to be properly diagnosed even when exhibiting many of the signs and symptoms, including blanching and sensitivity to touch, which increasingly worsened over time and with each new trauma.

The only part of the process that went reasonably well was applying and receiving a Social Security Disability rating. What happened to me should not happen to anyone ever. This applies to an even larger extent with our military members who are putting their own lives at risk for us.

In the matter before this Committee, I am representing the Power of Pain Foundation in its effort to speak for Active Duty soldiers and veterans who are going through many of the same issues I have gone through as a civilian.

I am here to urge the Advisory Committee to recommend that RSD be added to the Schedule of Diagnosis for which disability awards are granted by the Veterans Administration.

According to a 2006 survey taken by the American Pain Foundation, 54 percent of returning war veterans with chronic pain are diagnosed with Polytrauma or Causalgia, both military code for RSD. Based on data from RSDHope of America, Reflex Sympathetic Dystrophy Syndrome Association, For Grace, the American Pain Foundation, the National Institute of Neurological Disorders and Strokes, there are millions of patients with RSD across the United States and, of course, the world.

The high estimate is six million Americans. There are also more than 50,000 new cases diagnosed each year in the United States. Until more research is done and more doctors are educated in the correct diagnosis and treatment of RSD, it will be impossible to determine the exact count.

RSD is a progressive neurological condition that typically begins after an injury. In fact, it was first discovered among wounded soldiers over 150 years ago. RSD has been documented since the Civil War under many different names.

It was first studied by Dr. Weir Mitchell. In October 1864, Dr. Mitchell and his associates, G.R. Moorhouse and W.W. Keen, published a book called Gunshot Wounds and Other Injuries of Nerves. This book reveals some of the symptoms and signs first observed at Turner Alne Hospital for Nervous Diseases in Philadelphia.

RSD can affect the trunk, arms, legs and internal organs. It can be body wide or in one or more extremities. RSD was first discovered in the 19th century with severe, chronic pain and other symptoms, such as swelling, excessive sweating, and changes in skin color and temperature.

The same collection of symptoms that were true to RSD then are part of the condition today. As we gain a better understanding through research, modern science has added new symptoms to the list.

Mitchell's description of burning pain and a red-hot file rasping the skin are words RSD patients still connect with today. Mitchell first used the term "Causalgia," which means the burning pain, when describing his patients' symptoms. It was right on the money then, and it is still in the present day.

Since Mitchell named this condition Causalgia, there have been over 20 named designations. Some of them include Polytrauma; Reflex Neurovascular Dystrophy, RND; Algoneurodystrophy; Sudeck's Atrophy; Regional Pain Syndrome; Complex Regional Pain Syndrome, CRPS;

Reflex Sympathetic Dystrophy, RSD; Shoulder-Hand Syndrome; Post Traumatic Dystrophy; Painful Post Traumatic Dystrophy; Painful Post-Traumatic Osteoporosis; and Transient Migratory Osteoporosis.

According to the McGill pain scale, the rating system used internationally to measure pain, RSD rates worse than cancer, childbirth with no medication, amputation, and all others on the list.

No matter the name, RSD is the worst pain condition known to man, and those of us with it would agree totally.

A greater understanding came during World War I. In the early 1920s, German physicians began a focus on Causalgia under the name Sudeck's Atrophy. Researcher Benisty described movement disorders, such as tremors relating to Causalgia. Both Benisty and Tinel detailed peripheral nerve injures and Causalgia and a possible connection to a sympathetic nervous system origin.

Other doctors provided additional research on symptoms of RSD such as glossy skin, skin temperature changes, and reflex involvement. Some later doctors, such as Purves-Steward, Evans and Carter, used Mitchell as a reference when working on research in patients.

Mitchell's findings were also the basis of research by French doctors to further finding the origin of RSD. Although German physicians described Causalgia, they did not use the term, and this may be because Mitchell's findings were not translated into German. In all, RSD has been studied around the world by many researchers, scientists and physicians. They have come to many of the same conclusions as to the symptoms that RSD causes.

In 1983, Dr. Poplawski from Canada published a study about the long-term outcome of patients with RSD. He showed that RSD diagnosed in the first two years has a chance of successful treatment in 90 percent of patients, and after two years, each year drops the percentage of the success significantly.

Other doctor's say within the first six to nine months is the window for remission. A study by the International Association for the Study of Pain recommends that psychological intervention be initiated for patients experiencing pain for more than two months.

One study evaluating quality of life issues among patients with RSD reported that the greatest interruption in daily life was related to activities of daily living.

In the past 20 years, several double-blind studies reported the effectiveness of IV-Ketamine infusions as a noninvasive treatment for RSD. The FDA-approved drug insert supports the safety of Ketamine. Ketamine has a wide margin of safety. Several instances of unintentional administration of overdoses of Ketamine, up to ten times the normal dose usually required, have been followed by prolonged but complete recovery.

RSD specialists and the FDA work together to create a protocol for the administration of IV Ketamine for RSD patients. Ketamine is being used at doses approved by the FDA to treat and control pain due to RSD. Some insurance companies might try to argue that the FDA did not approve Ketamine to treat RSD; however, the FDA gave no specific medical condition as an indication for the drug.

No medication has ever been approved by the FDA officially to treat RSD. Yet, insurance companies routinely cover most medications to treat this neurological disorder.

The off-label use of drugs is common in the United States and Canada. In January 2009, the Canadian government recognized escalating doses of IV-Ketamine on an outpatient basis as a treatment for RSD.

Next up is going to be a video that aired in September that tells about my story and how I went into remission.

[Short video presentation.]

MS. INGLE: In April 2009, I was diagnosed with full body RSD. My RSD has spread from a brachial plexus nerve injury to full body RSD because of the treatments and complications I underwent based on doctor recommendations. The lack of understanding when it comes to diagnosing and treatment of RSD in the medical community is causing major disabilities and long-term issues that are more costly over the life of the patient's treatment.

This is one of the top reasons there is a lack of understanding as to the severity and disabilities that RSD causes patients. The good news is a group of RSD specialists and researchers have developed a protocol that is a noninvasive IV procedure. In December 2009, I underwent this procedure in Drexel Hospital and have received five follow-up boosters to maintain the remission effects of the initial IV inpatient Ketamine procedure.

The initial treatment and follow-up boosters are administered through IV therapy, similar to IV chemotherapy treatments. There's a cocktail of medications given--the Ketamine, Clonidine, Versed, Ativan, and a nausea medication.

Ketamine is the medication that actually works to put the patient into remission. The other medications are used to take away the side effects of the Ketamine such as hallucinations, vomiting and anxiety.

"Subanesthetic doses help but do not cure patients," Dr. Schwartzman said. Only the coma doses have cured patients.

Another specialist, Dr. Harbut, said of his Subanesthetic approach: "I believe this area of work is going to become and stay extremely exciting for years to come because of the relief it has and will bring to the care for intractable CRPS."

The difference between remission and a cure is how long relief asks after treatment. There are other noninvasive treatments that are available, such as hyperbaric oxygen therapy, massage therapy, sympathetic nerve blocks, tens unit, and topical pain patches.

Relief from these other treatments is not as effective in pain reduction nor as long lasting as IV-Ketamine treatments have shown to be over the years of research and studies. Still, use of these noninvasive treatment modalities is important before turning to invasive treatment such as spinal cord stimulators and Sympathectomies.

As I well know, any new trauma or insult to the body can increase the spread and severity of RSD. Although I'm in remission, I have to be careful physically because any new trauma can take me out of remission. This includes something that others would be fine with such as physical therapy, exercises with weights.

This everyday activity can be seen as a trauma or insult to the body, reversing the benefits of Ketamine, and as I found out on Saturday, also, a hard handshake can do the same.

According to recent studies, the survival rate for those wounded in Iraq and Afghanistan is better than 90 percent. This is due, in part, to improved body armor, surgical care deployed on the war front and rapid evacuation of the wounded to hospitals on aircraft equipped with advanced life support systems.

The flip side of this medical triumph is an unusually high percentage of soldiers returning home from Iraq and Afghanistan in pain. Because of the types of physical activities a soldier performs, injuries to multiple body parts and body systems increases the chance that veterans will experience chronic pain of some kind.

The average age of servicemen and women has increased to the age of 33.4 years. This too increases the risk for experiencing chronic pain. Several studies have found that nearly half of all veterans seeking care from the Veterans Administration report some degree of pain.

As we've heard today, RSD is not always permanently disabling. More often than not, it is disabling or progresses to a stage of permanent disability due to the lack of early diagnosis and proper treatment. The Veterans Administration should give their Disability Rating Board the authority to bestow a disability rating to veterans who suffer with RSD in order to decide their level of disability benefits after meeting a set standard of criteria.

The Social Security Administration uses the International Association for the Study of Pain criteria with the most recent revised version from 2004.

The disability rating should be based on documented, objective neurological testing and evaluation of subjective reporting to be supported by evidence and information collected on the Pain Disability Index.

Our veterans deserve benefits for RSD when it leads to disabling pain and other symptoms that interfere with work quality and activities of daily living.

Once again, thank you very much for allowing me to present to you today.

[Applause.]

CHAIRMAN SCOTT: Well, let me start off by asking if there are Committee members with questions or comments about Ms. Ingle's presentation?

The one thing I didn't quite catch, Ms. Ingle, is your initial injury was just to the shoulder; was that what it was?

MS. INGLE: Yes. I started with a whiplash injury, a brachial plexus nerve injury, and I was complaining of shoulder pain. My face, shoulder and neck were burning, and from that, they did a lot of tests. None of them showed anything was wrong, but they started doing a shoulder surgery. They took out my rib. There was complications. I had to have a lung surgery. I had to have my rib surgery again.

I had tumors grow in my mouth that had to be removed. I have bone deterioration in my face, and so on and so forth. I've had two kidney stones and they hurt a lot less than RSD does.

CHAIRMAN SCOTT: So the overtreatment or the erroneous treatment of your initial injury was what generated the syndrome; is that right?

MS. INGLE: I had the syndrome from the brachial plexus nerve injury, the whiplash, and the additional surgeries exacerbated it. Any new trauma can make it spread or progress.

CHAIRMAN SCOTT: Okay. All right. Yes?

DR. BLANCK: I'm fascinated by the Ketamine treatment and the cocktails, and that's a very, very positive thing obviously.

MS. INGLE: It is. I was in a wheelchair ten months ago. I wasn't able to walk. So I am doing very well, although I, like I said, I was injured on Saturday, and I'm starting to feel the burn come back and some of my Dystonia and sweating and stuff, discoloration.

DR. BLANCK: So you'll need another treatment?

MS. INGLE: So I need another one when I get home. This week I'll be checking with the doctor to see when I can get one.

DR. BLANCK: I guess the question then is how widespread is this being used? Is it pretty generally used at pain clinics?

MS. INGLE: No, it's not. The inpatient version that I underwent, I was a on a two-year waiting list to get into see the doctor that's doing it. There's one doctor that's doing the inpatient version that I did that put me into remission.

I did inpatient because I am full-body RSD. It affects my heart and intestines now. And I was in the hospital for seven days. The first day they titrate you up to the maximum allowed dose in the United States, and you're there for five days, and then the last day they titrate you back down.

After that, you have four mandatory boosters that are outpatient, and those are being done by some doctors in the United States, but there's not very many. So it's hard to get in to get those done.

DR. BLANCK: And then the follow-up, which I don't expect you would know, is the military and is the VA using these treatments?

MS. INGLE: Dr. Harbut back in 2003, it was reported that he was doing them at a VA hospital in I believe--do you know--in Georgia, I believe, there's a base there that they were doing them. I tried to find research when I was looking to prepare for today, and I couldn't find any additional information after 2003.

DR. BLANCK: I believe my information is that Walter Reed was using the Ketamine on a protocol in selected patients, I would expect for RSD.

Yeah, the VA Hospital is hooked up with Eisenhower Medical Center in Augusta that I believe is using it.

MS. INGLE: Georgia.

DR. BLANCK: Also Medical College of Georgia.

MS. INGLE: Right.

MS. TURNER LOTT: Thank you for your presentation. What was the date of the onset of the RSD after your injury? Approximate?

MS. INGLE: Within four days, the burning started.

MS. TURNER LOTT: Four days.

MS. INGLE: Within four days. I had the discoloration, the swelling that had demarcation. You could see exactly where the swelling stopped, and from that swelling, they did testing and said that I had thoracic outlet syndrome, which is when nerves or blood flow can't get through, and so that's when they decided they were going to take out my rib, and thoracic outlet syndrome is a secondary syndrome that can be brought on by RSD or it can stand alone on its own.

MS. TURNER LOTT: How soon were you diagnosed with RSD?

MS. INGLE: It took almost three years. I was diagnosed in May of 2005, and my accident was September 2002. I saw over 40 doctors before I was diagnosed properly, and in the last eight years, I've seen over a hundred medical professionals.

MS. TURNER LOTT: You did not have any surgery after the RSD was diagnosed; is that correct?

MS. INGLE: That's correct.

MS. TURNER LOTT: All right. And are the anesthesiologists, are they the ones who are administering the injections, the infusions?

MS. INGLE: The IV infusions. Dr. Schwartzman is a Neurologist.

MS. TURNER LOTT: Neurologist.

MS. INGLE: In Arizona, the doctor who is doing my boosters is an Anesthesiologist.

MS. TURNER LOTT: Do you know the projected time that these treatments can last?

MS. INGLE: Well, technically, they could last a long time. If you don't have any new injuries or insults to your body, you could go with no pain for a very long time, to the rest of your life.

I have gone out of remission twice. Once was because I stepped on something and it impaled the bottom of my foot, and I also got tetanus from that, and so I had to have a booster for that and then I burnt my hand on a coffee burner, and that caused it, and then Saturday when my hand got crushed.

MS. TURNER LOTT: Thank you.

CHAIRMAN SCOTT: Other questions for Ms. Ingle?

MR. BATTAGLIA: I don't have a question for you, and I really commend you on your presentation here today, but I would like to suggest that we have some follow-up on this here with the VA to find out what it is doing on the IV-Ketamine.

CHAIRMAN SCOTT: Okay. All right. Well, at this point, since all three presenters are in the room, does anybody have any follow-up they want to make with Dr. Moskovitz, Colonel Strand or Ms. Ingle?

And again, I've invited Colonel Strand to join us tomorrow for the presentation by the, on the VA-DoD collaboration, and if Dr. Moskovitz or Ms. Ingle have any interest in that, you're welcome to attend it as well.

If not--yes, go ahead, Charlie.

MR. BATTAGLIA: I just have one question for Dr. Moskovitz and Colonel Strand on here as to whether or not they--I didn't hear any mention of the IV-Ketamine from either one of you. I'm wondering if you're fully aware of this?

DR. MOSKOVITZ: Yes. The issue of Ketamine infusion--Ketamine is an NMDA antagonist. An NMDA is neurotransmitter. Dr. Schwartzman, Bob Schwartzman from Drexel, is one of chief theorists and proponents of Ketamine infusion therapy. It was begun clinically in

Germany, and they are no longer doing it now. There is a clinic just over the border in Monterrey, Mexico.

Because of the controversy surrounding Ketamine infusion, unfortunately, control trials of Ketamine are not available. It has been used clinically on an open label, uncontrolled basis, and usually reserved for people with total body RSD, the most severe and refractory sorts.

The results can be highly dramatic, but the most intensive therapy requires a five-day coma. Literally, people are put into an ICU setting, an intensive care unit setting, and put to sleep for five days. The complication rate is--major complication rate is about 20 percent. There has been one fatality in an older person with secondary health impairments, who was so distressed and miserable with his CRPS that he took a great risk for the potential of getting relief from his pain, and unfortunately his cardiac impairments were too great and he died of complications.

Although everyone is severely distressed by such an event, this was a choice by someone who was seriously suffering the pain and distress of this disease.

Low intensity, outpatient use of Ketamine is increasingly popular, and anesthesiologist and pain managers are jumping on it like a robin on a worm because of the potential for benefit. It is not always successful, and Ms. Ingle's case is a heartening example of success, but it is not always successful.

And it is not the first choice among most pain managers because of the risks. There are adverse effects of Ketamine, but it does have potential, and it is under study. It is probably a downstream effect.

That is the current thinking is that, that the mechanism of disease is higher in the cascade of immunochemistry, and that the effects of the immunochemical impairment is on the synapse where the NMDA is affected by microglia and astrocytes so that the Ketamine doesn't actually get to the source of the disease, but gets at a downstream effect.

But it's like pushing the odometer button. It sort of resets the odometer to zero, but then the odometer is cranking up. True cures are probably an unrealistic expectation, but control of the disease, that's fine. If we can get there, that would be a great achievement.

COLONEL STRAND: I'd like to add that I've been prescribed an ointment of sorts that contains Ketamine, and it's not useful for the constant type of burning pain that I experience, but it helps with the wasp type stinging pains. I've had a few here today. But it seems to numb the area and to calm down that. It usually happens when I'm under stress or something like that, but it only lasts about an hour maximum, and then you can't use it constantly. I wish I could.

I'd just bathe in the stuff, but it's pretty powerful, and it does have a numbing effect when I'm at my worst. When I inquired, when I heard, of course, when you find out you got RSD, you Google online, and you find out everything you can about it, and you get in contact with support groups, and I found about the Ketamine and went to my pain management doctors, and I've had three in the military, and they're unfamiliar with the treatment. As such, they're not willing to do it. They want to get you out of the military and turn you over to the VA.

I called the VA. They said no, we don't do that either, and so we're kind of at a loss. It's apparently expensive and time consuming and everything else, and if you multiply that by the number of people with RSD, unless this becomes a standard within the VA hospitals, or they have this treatment available for everybody, it's going to be very, very difficult to get treatment.

The same with hyperbaric oxygen therapy. I'm working with another gentleman, who was just--I mentioned earlier--in the Navy, who was diagnosed with RSD, and he has been begging and pleading to get hyperbaric oxygen therapy because you'll grab any straw you can if it can provide some level of relief. And they said that due to the expense of this treatment, it would not available to him.

DR. BLANCK: Just for your information, Eisenhower and the VA in Augusta with Medical College of Georgia, and I believe that's what you alluded to where they're doing that, using Ketamine, also has a hyperbaric chamber for whatever use that is.

COLONEL STRAND: And what you'll hear from the representatives is it's not a treatment for RSD.

Therefore, they're not going to do it. That's a typical answer we will get when we ask about those types of things. There's a very specific list of things that they will use HBOC treatment for, and RSD is not on the list. So if you can help us get that done, maybe that could help.

MS. TURNER LOTT: Doctor, what is the most common adverse effect of Ketamine?

DR. MOSKOVITZ: Hallucinations are common. The Midazolam and sedative cocktails minimize that, but, and also just cognitive therapy, pointing out to people before they start the program that bad dreams and hallucinations are common. Ketamine started its life as an anesthetic, a dissociative anesthetic, and people retained their reflexive protective mechanisms for swallowing and breathing so that they appeared to have all of their maintenance, vegetative functions intact, but are just out of it, and this makes it a fairly safe anesthetic for young people, people who have sustained trauma who need acute care where a period of being without food or water before the anesthetic is impossible. Open fractures and the like.

Unfortunately, these cognitive impairments intervene. But if you just tell somebody to expect that, then the disturbing nature of the dreams goes away, and they are short-lived. Did you have that, Ms. Ingle?

MS. INGLE: I did have a few hallucinations, but they were all positive and happy.

DR. MOSKOVITZ: Oh, good.

MS. INGLE: And I don't remember any of them. People have reported back to me. I don't--afterwards it's a blank memory.

DR. MOSKOVITZ: In the Ketamine coma work, there are--very frequently people had urinary tract infections because they required bladder intubation; respiratory infections. Pneumonia is not uncommon. So that the five-day coma treatments are quite troublesome that way.

Otherwise, there don't appear to be a lot of serious adverse effects.

MS. TURNER LOTT: How long do the hallucinations last? Are we talking about just during the treatment or three months or two years?

DR. MOSKOVITZ: I can't give you--I'm not an expert in this treatment. I don't do it. I don't administer it myself. My understanding is that they are short-lived, but once in awhile they'll come back as flashbacks. Again, cognitive therapy seems to minimize that. It's rather simple.

MS. TURNER LOTT: Did you say there are no clinical trials?

DR. MOSKOVITZ: There are no controlled clinical trials. There is something called the Ketamine Coma Study, which is run by Dr. Schwartzman and Tony

Kirkpatrick from Florida. It's basically a show-and-tell study. It's a sequence of patients. I regret to report that I've heard about more failures than seems to be reported in what's out there.

There are a few papers that appear in the literature on the effects of Ketamine, but they're basically anecdotal studies, and it's unfortunate, that there isn't funding. It's a very expensive process. It's privately funded by individuals, and there has been a lot of conflict about how to get funding for people who need Ketamine treatment.

MS. INGLE: I would to say that Medicare does pay for inpatient Ketamine and Ketamine boosters, and a lot of the insurance companies are now paying so--

CHAIRMAN SCOTT: Okay. Are there other comments or questions at this time?

Well, as I had mentioned earlier, in the case of all three of you, once we get into this a little bit deeper with the VA, we may very well ask for a follow-up e-mail, phone call or visit, and understand that for the two of you traveling is not easy, and we'll try to work around that.

But I'd like to thank all three of you. It's been extremely enlightening, very helpful. Certainly speaking for myself, it certainly increased my understanding of the entire and complex nature of the syndrome, and we will take it up with the VHA and the VBA sides of VA in sequence, and see what sort of a resolution we can come up with about making it easier or simpler to diagnose and evaluate.

So I'd like to thank all three of you. Very much appreciate it, and also appreciate the very good handouts. These are very useful for future reference material.

So with that, Committee members, let's take a ten minute break, and then we'll reconvene and take up the next issue, which is the update on the Musculoskeletal Work Group.

[Whereupon, a short break was taken.]

Ketamine Infusion Information

This is based on Barby's treatments as well as many other patient references. Keep in mind that every patient is different and your doctor is the one to determine what will work best for you.

Pre K-Infusion
1. Testing
   a. Laboratory
   b. Cardiac
   c. Psychological evaluation

Hospital-based infusions
1. Five-day in-patient stay
   a. An intravenous (iv) line is inserted
   b. Dosing starts at 20mg of Ketamine per hour, which is increased by 5mg increments to a maximum of 40mg per hour
   c. Clonidine, 0.1 mg (per FDA)
   d. Lorazepam (Ativan®), 1-to-2 mg, for any dysphoria or hallucinations
   e. Other medications are utilized to treat such problems as nausea and vomiting, headache etc.

Outpatient protocol
1. Initial 10 day outpatient care
   a. Five days on, 2 off, five days on
   b. 70mg to 200mg of Ketamine per day in titrating doses over the 10 days and then start the outpatient booster program

c. Most patients are given 2 mg of Midazolam and sleep through the procedure

d. Other medications are given as needed for side effects such as nausea and headache

Booster Protocol

1. Following discharge from the hospital or 10 day outpatient care, patients enroll in an outpatient infusion booster program

   a. The booster program consists of two consecutive outpatient treatments a week every other week for one month, then two consecutive treatments one month later, then two consecutive treatments at three months.

   b. Outpatient visits are then monthly, or at 3-month intervals. This is done in two or more consecutive days. Exact protocol depends on the patient and varies at times.

   c. Barby's outpatient dose of Ketamine is 200mg each day.

COME WHAT MAY…

… AND SO IT IS!

ReMission Possible

Yours, If You Choose To Accept It

www.ingramcontent.com/pod-product-compliance
Lightning Source LLC
Chambersburg PA
CBHW050128280326
41933CB00010B/1297